NORDIC WISDOM

KARITA AALTONEN

I Survived:

A Nordic Woman's Guide to Healing from Cancer

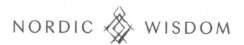
NORDIC WISDOM

© Karita Aaltonen
© Nordic Wisdom, 2021

ISBN: 978-952-7449-00-4

Based on the author's book Uskalla Parantua,
published in Finland by Viisas Elämä, 2017

English translation by Elisa Wulff
Book design and illustrations by Jaana Virronen
Photography by Elise Kulmala

To find out more about our authors, books, and courses visit nordicwisdom.com.
Here you will find the option to sign up for our newsletter.
Discover that one thing that changes everything.

CONTENTS

PREFACE

Who am I? I am a mother, a wife, a friend, a caregiver, an activist, an organizer, a yoga teacher. I love to laugh and make jokes so dark other people are afraid to laugh. I love to share tea and cinnamon buns and coffee with friends. I love sitting outside and watching the Finnish summertime midnight sun.

I am also one of the longest living survivors of Glioblastoma Multiforme grade IV, the most fatal and aggressive brain cancer known. It is almost always terminal. 25% of glioblastoma patients survive more than one year, and only 5% of patients survive five years. Less than 1% survive beyond five years.

I'm beyond nine years now.

I would like to tell you my story, in my own words, and as I have experienced it.

This is not just my story. This is also a story about my whole family, friends, and loved ones, as cancer touches so many people around us. This is a story about despair, fear, and sadness. Above all, this is a story about perseverance, tenacity, hope, and the power of the mind, and finally, about understanding.

The modern Nordic approach to living well is this: anything that works. Although deeply appreciated, our own traditions and beliefs are not literal or metaphorical hills we are willing to die on. Us Finns respect nature, silence, time spent not working, regular weekly relaxation (sauna!), our folk wisdom, medicinal herbs, etc. At the same time, we embrace other ancient practices, such as yoga, traditional Chinese medicine, or Ayurveda. We remain open to other ideas. We try new things, and if they are beneficial, incorporate them into our lives. This is the very definition of flexibility. We do not stand in our own way.

I hope this book provides hope and helps you trust in your own healing potential. I hope this book will help many people struggling with cancer or other diseases who wish to take responsibility for their own health and healing. I promise you are not alone, whatever your circumstances.

While this book is a story of my own cancer journey, it is also about all the people and tools that have contributed to my healing process. However, I must emphasize that I am still on this journey.

This journey has no destiny. – Karita ♡

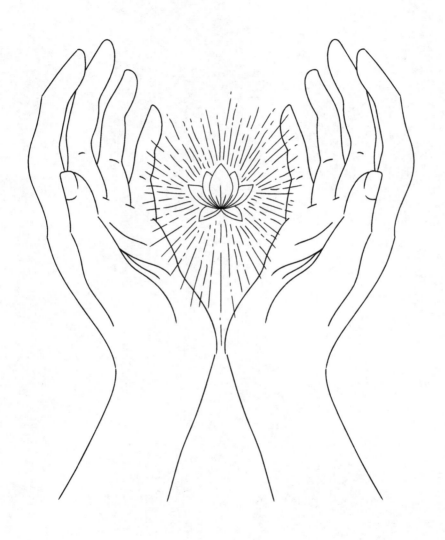

MY NEW FRIEND

On Valentine's Day in 2012, I found out I had incurable brain cancer.

"I'm sure this is nothing, but....." I cringe as I detail to my doctor the curious symptoms I'd experienced during the last six months: legs suddenly giving out underneath me, hands unable to grasp a drinking glass, strange sensations like the feeling of being inside a vacuum and unaware of things going on around me, an eerie sense of someone beside me—I'd reach out to touch them and there'd be nothing there.

I know how weird they sound, and also I'm fine.

I believed I was fine. This was obviously a waste of my time. I have always been healthy. Always! Never been at the hospital, never sick. I did not feel any pain. I felt "healthy" but at the same time I knew all the weird symptoms I'd had in the past six months. Here I am, taking an appointment away from someone who actually needs to see a doctor. Earlier in the morning I considered canceling my appointment, but then felt embarrassed to cancel so late. So there I was.

The doctor looks at me, hard. Too hard. And, to my horror, sends me upstairs to take an MRI. Immediately. It could not wait. My What-If Generator starts working overtime. I'm struck by a cascade of thoughts, fear, horror: Losing my children. Will I die of this? When will I die? Can I be a mother anymore? Endless alternatives came to mind of what could be wrong: ALS, MS, cancer. No, no, no!

I lay down inside the magnetic tube and they place an iron cage over my head. "Stay perfectly still," I'm instructed. Time stretches thin and as I lie there, listening to the strange poundings of the machine working, I will myself to think about other things. Laundry, picking up the kids, what I might make for dinner later. Anything but what might be wrong with me, or where I actually am. Time went from stretching to standing completely still.

The attending nurse will not meet my gaze. In fact, she even looks as though she is about to cry. "The doctor would like to see you immediately," she said in a grim tone.

The doctor also refuses to look me in the eye. He just stares at his computer screen and nervously rocks back and forth in their chair. We are both quiet. Then came the sentence that changed everything: "You have a malignant brain tumor."

Silence. Neither of us knew what to say. There we were,

sitting in silence, until the doctor quizzically raised his eyebrows: "Do you understand...?"

I did not. I will not. How could I understand, how could anyone! I had just turned from a fully healthy person into a fully sick one. Seriously ill. Terminally ill.

Tears rolled down my cheeks. My head felt empty and I was lost.

I most certainly do not have time to die! I have my children, my family, my job, my social life, my whole world! I'm needed every minute of every day. Dying is absolutely out of the question. Please, Karita, focus. Maybe I can will myself to be well. After all, I have many things I must do: Driving my kids to ice hockey practice, traveling around Finland for work, walking the dogs, house chores, meeting friends. So many things!! I can't die!

"Will you be able to drive back home?" the doctor asked. I nodded. Of course I was. I was a strong, independent woman, after all. Do they think I'm made of glass? I most certainly won't ask anyone for help. I mean, of course I could drive. What an odd question. Next they'll be asking if I need someone to help me put on my coat and walk me out!

Holding the diagnosis statement in my hand, I drive back home. I call my husband, Jussi, and burst into tears on the phone. I also call my friends, Johanna and Riina: "I know this is kind of sudden, but I think I have a brain tumor." Tactful, I know, but how else could you really say it?! There was nothing

I could say to preface, because I hadn't told my friends about my previous symptoms. I had known already, without accepting, I was ill. My cellphone started ringing while I was still driving. The hospital's chief neurosurgeon was on the other line and among the purely logistical things he said: "I'd like to give you one piece of advice. Don't look around online. Do not Google your diagnosis."

This was the best piece of advice I ever got. I didn't want to get on board with what I would have found by Googling. Grade 4 told me enough. It's very serious. Not knowing all the possibilities opened up a different set of possibilities - healing, scenarios of health and hope and positivity. I wouldn't have found any of that by Googling the diagnosis because there's nothing good about it online.

To this day, I have never typed the name of my diagnosis into Google: Glioblastoma Multiforme grade IV.

"Corpus callosum...on the left parietal lobe parasagitally to the central line and intra-axial expansion tangent to parietal dura...no skip lesion detected...basal nuclei level..." Whaaat? I didn't understand a word! Can you put it in words I can understand? Why talk to me like this? Just tell me what I need to know. Why do doctors have to be like this? I could feel my frustration rising and my head getting hot.

I'm great in a crisis, everyone says so. Even in my own crises, I can manage.

This was not different. I'm action-oriented. In my head, I started drawing up a list: what would I have to get done first, what next and so on.

The first thing I had to do was to cancel my hosting gigs. I didn't want to. I loved my work. I'd had my own company since 2000.

I started hiring temps for my gigs. This was the first time I told people outside of friends and family about the illness. I started to see how people were affected by what I told them. It touched them - they truly cared. My business partners broke out of the business character and their humanity came through. I realized whoever hears about my situation will be affected by it. At first I thought this was just my thing I'm going through alone. It was hard to recieve their responses and feel the great compassion they felt for me. I felt that my illness touched – and was going to touch – a large group of people.

My parents were cross-country skiing at their friend's cottage in Lapland. We decided we would not tell them about the disease while they were still on vacation. We took our time on how to address it with the children. At the time, Rene was eight and Nooa was five. "Let's make a plan on how to move forward", I told Jussi.

As they say, the best laid plans, etc. Despite the plans we made, Jussi called my parents two days later. I could not make myself call them. My mother answered her cellphone while on the skiing trip. We agreed that my parents would come straight to our home from their vacation and we would calmly discuss the topic among family. My sister, Kikka, and my good friend Riina also came over. We made coffee, someone brought pastries. It was all very normal, except instead of talking about the weather, or how frustrating it is when our boss is curt with us, we discussed my brain tumor.

I had never considered my own death. When it crossed my mind now, I quickly shifted my focus back to the world of the living. I wanted to live. I was not looking for a life of luxury; I'm satisfied with my own interesting life. There was a lot to do, courses to take, yoga classes, taking the dogs for walks, hosting gigs, and dinners with friends and families. All so wonderful and normal.

I just wanted things to be normal again.

Keeping our day-to-day as normal as possible was something we agreed on.

We told the children about my disease in a casual way. After all, they were too young to grasp the severity of the whole situation. We told the children that a "lump" had been found in mommy's head. We didn't use the word cancer or tumor in front of the kids. It felt less severe to call it a lump that just needs to be cut out. We told them mommy would go to the hospital where surgeons would make her okay. We said that everything was just fine. Sometimes, I wonder if we were also telling ourselves that. What would it be like, if we all talked to each other that way—in a kind of gentle reassuring tone?

"The tumor is operable". Finally, some good news! The operation was scheduled to take place on April 12th, 2012, Nooa's birthday.

Well, this year's celebration was going to be pretty different from any previous celebrations.

During that spring, while I waited, the thought why me never crossed my mind. I mean, I did think why it had to be me of all people. There has to be some sort of a greater meaning in all of this, some kind of a lesson to learn, I told myself. I was absolutely certain. I knew this new friend (my tumor) had come to teach me something. I did not know what exactly that was going to be, but I found the idea exciting. This kept my curiosity up, kept me open, the great mystery of Discovery was yet to unfold before me and I was here for it!

I refused to keep my illness a secret. I told people honestly and openly about what was going on. In my family, people didn't talk about negative things. But I didn't want to be like that. It was very clear from the beginning I wouldn't stay quiet about this. The Finnish way mostly is to be quiet, keep it within the family only. I defied that. For example, in Finland people don't talk about miscarriage or difficulty in getting pregnant. I didn't get why you can't talk about it because I've always been against stupid rules in general. Why can't someone just say, "I can't get pregnant. Fuck, this is hard!"

More recently, people in Finland do talk more openly about cancer than back then. When people talk about their issues, they get help more easily. Why don't Finns talk openly about problems? I think we're a quiet folk historically, more introverted, and don't want to burden others with our problems. Shame is real in Finland.

Finns are honest and direct but not always open about their problems or what's seen as personal. We don't want to burden the other person. We want to spare the other person from the weight of our issues, it's a matter of being polite and considerate, in our minds.

No matter how I put it, it came across as blunt. "Please don't be alarmed by this but...I have a brain tumor." That is it. That is how you break it to people. In Finland we don't do small talk. When people ask "How are you?", you tell them how you are. When I met a friend at a grocery store, she smiled and said, "Hi! How are you?". And I, not doing well, couldn't reply with "Good, how are you?". Instead I said: "Please don't be alarmed by this but... I have a brain tumor." This is how I told every friend, acquaintance, loved one, relative. I told everyone there is no reason to keep this a secret. And it did not take long until almost everyone knew it. Loved ones, familiar people, distant acquaintances, and complete strangers. It was all for the better. If I got the chance to disclose, no one could write the scene for me. Controlling the narrative felt extremely empowering, and I thought about how this could translate to other parts of my life.

I knew the surgery would take six to seven hours, I knew my body needs to be strong so it can endure. I needed to strengthen my body and mind. Vitamins, "my witch drinks", spirulina, chlorella, antioxidants, smoothies. The mind has to be strong and trust that everything will go fine. I prepared by putting the "problem" into a framework of "challenge." I did not use the word "problem."

I considered who could help me prepare for the surgery, which would be mentally and physically challenging, no matter the circumstances. The only person that popped into my mind was Heikki Harju, a wellness coach I had met the previous summer at an event I was hired to MC. He was the only person I knew in my city from the health community - which at the time I wasn't part of - I knew had knowledge of nutrition, and the impact of mind to your health. He focused on how to use one's mind correctly, or for healing. Heikki is friendly and approachable and has wonderful warm energy, so I knew only good things could come out of meeting him. This was the beginning of gathering my people around me. People who contribute good vibes and positivity, and don't bring negativity, fear, worry into the situation. I wrote Heikki an email telling him about my illness and coming operation, and asked him for help. You never know who might be willing to help unless you ask. Heikki's response was lovely and encouraging:

There are many things in life that other people would refer to as "problems." This is known as negativity. Other people are more positive and call these things "challenges." That is a better starting point in life. Life is what we perceive it to be. Our interpretations of the world shape our reality into the very thing we see it as. Letting go of these interpretations allows us to see all problems and challenges, and the whole life itself, as an opportunity.

Life is an opportunity. What do you want from it?

What do I want from life? From that premise we began building the pillars of my health before my first challenge—the surgery to remove the brain tumor. My body would have to be strong, strong enough to withstand the surgery, which was life-threatening. My mind would have to be strong enough to not shatter. I would have to trust that the whole procedure would go smoothly. I want to live, and live well.

Based on Heikki's instructions, I began adding a lot of antioxidants and medicinal herbs into my diet, including chaga mushrooms, conifer extract drink, lemon, fresh berries, green smoothies, and green powders. I started drinking a lot of clean water and using healthy types of salt. I collected pure spring water from nature. There's a website loydalahde.com ("find a well") where you can find springs near you. Some have pumps in place. Thus I could access natural clean water with no chemicals added like chlorine, iron etc. I started taking high-quality omega 3 fatty acids (which I had to discontinue using a month before the surgery due to an increased bleeding risk, just FYI!). Alkaline, alkaline, alkaline. All aiming to make my body as strong as possible to withstand the upcoming and unavoidable surgery day.

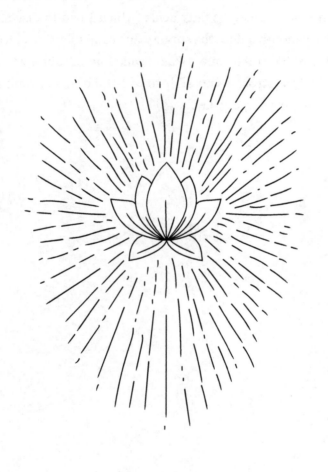

SURGERY DAY

I spent all spring preparing for the operation. Spring in Finland lasts for about three months before giving way to summer. Finland, the land of 100,000 lakes. The ice melts, the snow disappears, the rivers run full and fast. Everything blooms in such beauty and best of all, the sun returns from its own hibernation. You can feel the entire country stretching its stiff muscles and breathing a sigh of relief. Winter can't last forever, and never does, even if you can't remember what being warm outside feels like.

The feelings of defiance and perseverance grew in me, just like the leaves and buds of Finnish spring: this is just something I will have to push through! I wanted to get back to my own familiar, normal life. The life that I thought makes me happy. The mere idea of not being around to see my children grow up made me feel sick and sad. I was certainly not ready to die for a long, long time. No eternal winter for me.

The morning of surgery day arrived. All morning, I listened to the soundtrack of the Mamma Mia musical. I had songs like "Mamma Mia," "Winner Takes It All," "Honey Honey," and "What's The Name Of The Game" playing on full volume in my earphones. When a nurse came to tell me it was time to go to the operating room, I kept the earphones tightly in my ears. I did not want to panic. It was easier to listen to music. Jussi walked alongside me for as long as he was permitted and gave me well wishes for the surgery. He squeezed my hand. He looked at me tenderly. He was panicked but kept a stiff upper lip—he didn't want to break down in front of me. I could see I felt more peaceful than my husband or parents. The premedication might have contributed to my calmness—literal chill pills.

When you're ill, you still have more feeling of control than your loved ones. Throughout my illness journey, I had to trust my intuition and make my own choices. There was no peer support, because the condition is so rare. I had no one to talk to. But I had total control making these decisions, whereas loved ones didn't even have that. A really serious illness is an even bigger impact to your loved ones because they have zero control over it, they feel like outsiders, in a way, with the situation.

Jussi walked me as far through the hospital hallways as he was allowed to, until the nurse said, "You must stay here, you can't go further." After Jussi and I separated, I kept my eyes closed until I reached the operating table. I peeked through my lids to see what the operating room looked like. I swiftly closed my eyes again. I kept my eyes closed because it was such a scary situation to be taken to a surgery room where I'd never been. I didn't want to see other people or be seen, although of course they saw me. But it was easier to stay calm with my eyes closed.

As if by a miracle, I was able to consider the surgery as an interesting adventure– after all, this was my first time in a hospital, let alone in a major surgery. I guessed the room was full of heavy tools, I mean, they are cutting open my head. So I wanted not to see that. Instead, I focused on my breathing. I had seen other people panic in the hospital. I decided to stay in my own inner peace and calm.

I had already met my surgeon. Our meeting included going over the risks of the operation, so I knew it was considerably likely that something could go wrong. The slightest error, say, one millimeter in the wrong direction, could cause major, irreversible damage. In fact, this could even occur without any errors made by a surgeon, as it was almost impossible for the surgeon to know for certain which tissue was cancerous and which was healthy. The surgery was estimated to take between six and seven hours, after which I would be taken to the intensive care unit.

The nurse told me they would count to five....

One...
Two...
Three...
.....
......

When I woke up at the intensive care unit, my first thought was that at least I was alive. I was so happy I just wanted to cry. So happy to be alive. I thought of all the hundreds of people who were with me in this. This was something so big. Something was happening to me. I felt the change. I FELT more than I had ever felt in my past. I could cry and laugh at the same time. I was living and breathing! I could see wires or tubes attached to every part of my body. I even giggled to myself that they had turned me into some kind of bionic woman! All the devices made regular beeps and blips. A monitor surveyed my every heartbeat. I moved my fingers and toes slightly. Yes, I could sense a bit of movement. I also knew where I was and what time it was. I knew who I was. I was also insanely hungry and thirsty.

An intensive care nurse, Ulla, came over and sat down next to me. She was a short woman with red hair. Her eyes were full of empathy. Ulla looked me straight in the eyes and asked: "What planet are you from? No one is in such great shape when waking up after major brain surgery!" Without wanting to seem rude or demanding, but also beginning to unravel from hunger and thirst, I said as nicely as I possibly could. "Ulla, I'm going to faint unless you give me something to eat." Normally at this stage, right after a major operation, they will not give you any food, but Ulla saw my primitive anguish and gave in. I promised not to tell anyone. When she gave me yogurt and a bottle of water, I mentally fell to my knees and wept. You can't know this kind of gratitude unless you've experienced it yourself. Carbonated water has never, ever tasted as good.

"Okay, so now we can talk."

Ulla wanted to know how I could be so normal under the circumstances, right after waking up from general anesthesia. They had only just taken an endotracheal tube from out of my mouth. I told Ulla about Heikki who had given me good tips on how to prepare for the operation. I talked about how I had put my sodium balance in order, been taking vitamins and drinking antioxidant beverages. I had also been preparing mentally by thinking positively. I trusted that it would all work out. I truly trusted it!

I was given intravenous pain medicine, which allowed me to get through it all with fairly minor pains. At times, I asked for more drugs, and they always gave them to me. I was accompanied by a nurse at all times. And they were all very encouraging and supportive.

It's important to talk here about the healthcare system in Finland, as it differs heavily from the healthcare systems of other countries, particularly the US. There is free healthcare for everyone in Finland. Your status doesn't matter. You don't need insurance. All Finland residents are automatically insured by Finland. Everyone's guaranteed the same high, world-class level of healthcare - your behavior, background, nothing affects it.

Chemotherapy and the accompanying pharmaceuticals cost thousands of euros. In the US, it costs hundreds of thousands. Here, one week's dose of chemo drug costs 1500 euros and I was prescribed 12 weeks annually. I paid about 3e total per week. My epilepsy medications cost only a couple of euros too. Finland pays for them - the society does - that's why we pay taxes.

EQUALITY is so important. Healthcare and education are equally available and free for all. You pay nothing for going to high school, university, getting a PhD. You only buy the school books when past elementary school. Lunches (healthy food!) are free in elementary school, high school.

Money won't get you different service at a store or education in a school. Everyone gets the same. That's why in Finland it's a priority to keep the level of education, healthcare etc. very high because everyone will get it, including the rich and the lawmakers. It's in their interest to keep the quality very high. Because that's what they'll get, too.

After the operation, the surgeon in charge immediately called my husband, Jussi, telling him that the surgery had gone well and that I was alive. This phone call was truly unforgettable to Jussi, it was the most relief he'd ever felt in his life. Afterwards, Jussi told me he had been extremely nervous. During the surgery, he had paced back and forth in the hospital, for the whole 6 hours — panicking. After speaking with the surgeon Jussi immediately called my parents, who I am sure had been sitting by the phone, scared stiff.

I hoped they would let Jussi see me at the intensive care unit – preferably as soon as humanly possible. Like, YESTERDAY. It was such a relief to see a person who had been living by my side through it all. This was something we shared together. It was not just about me.

Jussi arrived at the same time as my surgeon to see how I was doing. At this point, my tumor was estimated as grade II or III based on a frozen section specimen. That was tolerable. Way better than the grade IV that they had originally assessed it as.

"We will get the final results once we receive a pathologist's statement in a few weeks," Dr. Tähtinen said.

The next day, I was transferred from the intensive care unit to a normal ward, where they could keep closely monitoring my recovery. The nurses gave me pain medication and, in the evenings, sleep medicine. They also offered me sedatives for anxiety, but I refused them, feeling that I did not need them. When there's been a big operation in the hospital, they automatically give you anxiety medicines to ease the recuperation. I had a certain calmness and didn't have panic-attack feelings. The drugs would have covered up my feelings. I wanted to go through it as it was, and not remove feelings from the equation.

I felt very much at home in the hospital. It's funny how quickly you start feeling "institutionalized." The outside world seems foreign, while you feel safe and taken care of at the hospital. Someone was tending to me at all times. There was a certain rhythm and schedule to everything. It felt safe. It was easy and quiet. All sounds felt loud and harsh to me. Food is prepared and brought to you. You don't have to do anything, except use the toilet. In fact, that was the most painful part of the whole week! The combination of anesthetics and other medications used during the surgery, plus staying completely still, made me all blocked up. Gross! Maybe TMI, but true. I asked the nurses for all kinds of remedies, and it took almost a week for things in that department to return to normal.

My friends came to visit me each day. The nurses teased me, saying they were glad I had the room to myself—such was the joyful laughter that went on there. At any given time, there might be ten women sitting on my bed, making jokes. We laughed tears of joy. At times, I had to hold back my amusement as laughing hurt my head during the first days after the surgery. I tried to laugh while staying as still as possible.

My childhood friends brought me scarves as gifts. All kinds of scarves, in all possible colors. We laughed at my childhood fantasy of being a farm matron wearing a scarf on her head and boots on her feet, taking care of cattle and sheep that would never be slaughtered but that would just run free and happy on a lawn, eating grass. Although I never became a farm woman, at least I would be able to wear those scarves now. My friends had also made me a card with multiple pages, full of our shared memories, encouraging phrases, and touching thoughts. They had really gone through a lot of trouble digging through old photographs of different parts of our lives. Photos from birthday parties in a dress blowing the candles on a cake, at music festivals, at parties dancing to Duran Duran.

All these wonderful, caring people.

My surgeon came to see me and casually said, "Of course, you'll lose your driving license now." The way he said it was monotone, as if he had just noted something as mundane as "Today, you'll be having vegetable soup for lunch." I felt as if he had just thrown a wet rag against my face. I'm sorry, what? What, what, what — and why? "You are at a major risk of having epileptic seizures. We're starting preventive medication for epilepsy now and you won't be able to drive for a year, minimum."

How was I going to be able to take my children to their hobbies, go to yoga classes, or visit downtown? It felt like a huge deal. Even though I had just gone through a major brain

surgery, I was worried about not being able to drive. No –
you are absolutely not going to take this from me! I was not
going to stand for it. And what was this talk about epilepsy,
anyway? I had a brain tumor, not epilepsy. I begged for more
careful examinations. I did not want to take medication "just
to be sure" and I refused to give up my driving license "in case
something might happen..."

The doctors promised to get back to it later, but I would
lose my license in any case.

It's easy to get used to hospital life. The days follow a familiar
pattern, which creates a sense of security. There's breakfast,
blood tests, waiting for doctor's rounds, lunch, visits from
friends, a nap, dinner, maybe listening to some music, an
evening snack, and sleep. And then it all starts again in the
morning, at seven o'clock...so safe and familiar. Lovely. I was
not ready to get back home yet. It was all so easy there at the
hospital. The outside world felt so unfamiliar. Nothing had
changed out there.

But for me, everything had changed.

When the doctor was making rounds, I always came up
with reasons why they should let me stay there a little longer. But these were real reasons: sounds did actually hurt my
head, it felt as if noise literally cut through my brain. It was
hard to imagine how I would be able to cope at home; after all,
what awaited me there were two children and two dogs and all

the normal hustle and bustle known as my everyday life.

Jussi brought green smoothies and vitamins to the hospital. I hid them in the drawer of my bedside table. I also hid some medications that I did not want to take—sleep medicine, anxiety drugs. I did take the pain medication because my head hurt so much after the operation. I seemed so well that they discharged me from the hospital on my sixth day there. I was sad to say goodbye to the wonderful nurses at the ward. I even missed my blue and pink hospital gowns. Now came the time to wear my regular clothes. To put on some mascara. Maybe even some lipstick.

A colorless ghost stared back at me in the mirror.

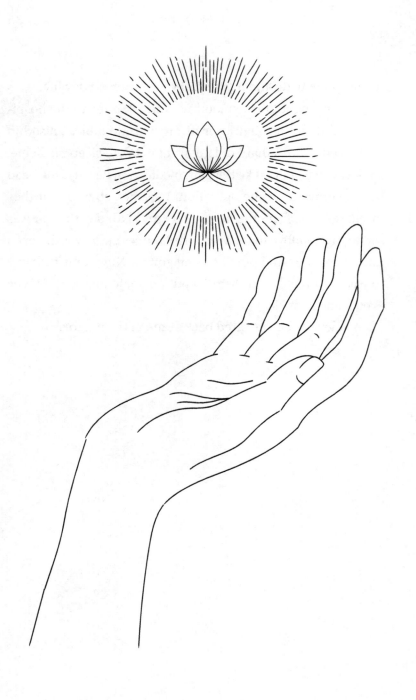

HOMECOMING

In all honesty, I was far from being ready to return home. I missed my children tremendously and felt I owed them for having been away. But, noises caused a splitting sensation in my head. I gripped my head and plugged my ears if noises were too loud. All my senses were on overload. My doctors had warned me of all of this, of course. I had to take it really slow, listening to my body. The first walk I took was to pick up the newspaper from our mailbox. Such a small trip took planning, and gathering of all my strength. Afterwards, I napped for three hours.

I spent two *long* weeks waiting for the pathologist's report. Finally, the surgeon called me and gave me the bad news: *I'm sorry to tell you that the tumor was grade III, called oligoastrocytoma.*

Grade III meant the recommended additional treatment included radiotherapy.

At this time, I was also referred for the evaluations for epilepsy I had asked for. I got a referral to an EEG, which measures the electric function and anomalies of the brain. Finding clear epileptiform patterns in the examination would mean that my medication would remain as previously prescribed. In the examination, the nurse put an EEG cap over my head, and I watched the flashing lights displayed before my eyes, without any idea of what was going on in my brain. I soon got a phone call of the results and they were also sent to me in writing at home:

> "In the EEG, on the left, slow activity is highlighted parieto-occipitally as a localized finding. On the left, profuse and prominent mu rhythm, probably stressed by the surgical wound on the skull, no undisputed epileptic activity. However, patient has experienced continuing moderate seizure symptoms, less than one minute in duration, seizures with numbness on the right extremities. Increasing Trileptal dosage to 300 mg 2 + 2."

They took my license away, indefinitely.

I'll let you in on the worst-kept secret of the modern world: taxi drivers have the best knowledge on pretty much *any* given topic. One taxi driver in the city of Nokia I got to know well said, "With your diagnosis, you're definitely eligible for shared rides." When you are sick in Finland you get free taxi service... if you are sick enough.

Before my illness I thought a taxi is a taxi, taking you from A to B. But in Finland, the taxi's biggest service is to take ill people and handicapped children to hospitals or between places they're going. The drivers hear a ton of medical information. They helped me get free rides to radiation and back, and of course to the hospital and back. I also got 18 free rides per month (with taxpayer money/Finnish healthcare) to go to yoga class, do shopping, take kids to their hobbies, and so on — it was up to me how to use them. In the hospital they hadn't talked about the taxi program so I didn't know. Additionally, I'd been told by a social worker that I *didn't* qualify. When I applied for the program, it turned out the driver was correct.

This taught me a few things:
1. always ask more than once
2. always ask more than one person
3. you'll never know who might have information that will prove helpful

The other passengers in the shared rides were elderly women and men, persons with disabilities, and children in need of other special support. I developed a great respect for taxi drivers, who really put their heart into what they did: they had energy to talk with the passengers, undoubtedly knowing how important this contact was to many of the older people—perhaps the only time they met another person during the day. I also had great admiration for those who always found time to ask the children how they were doing and talk with them. The young children were often nervous about the rides. Looking at them, you could often see the children had to be "big girls and boys" and cope with a lot more than their neurotypical peers who have no idea what special needs and disabled children cope with on a daily basis. These children had to keep a brave face. There were little children who go by taxi everywhere because they were disabled, maybe blind, in wheelchair. They had to act older than they are to cope with the stress of being taken by taxi to places, in a taxi with many other kids as well.

Sometimes it feels wonderful to be quiet. The taxi drivers could always sense whether you wanted to talk or stay silent. Talking about my illness with them came naturally, perhaps because they had so much experience in giving rides to sick people. In some way, I felt guilty for appearing so normal while still getting these paid-for taxi rides. I felt I had to keep convincing others of how sick I actually was, that it was something I had to prove.

During this period of radiotherapy, Aarni Kuorikoski, a TV producer, called me and asked me to participate in the Life for Children TV show produced by the Association of Friends of the University Children's Hospital charity organization. They were looking for someone to interview the families of pediatric patients, families with a severely ill child. These children often had cancer. Without giving it a second thought, I said yes—I was definitely in.

I was given a list of families and the illnesses they were affected by, and started preparing questions for them. I was able to organize my work so that I always had time to have radiotherapy either before or after the interviews.

I could never have imagined doing this without my personal experience. Meeting the families required huge emotional capacity, especially the sick children. Pema Chodron, a well known Tibetan Buddhist, talks about how we can only be with others to the degree with which we can be with ourselves. Somehow, I felt my own illness had given me a newfound strength to stay present. Still, it was not always easy. There were times when I could not control myself and wept—for instance, when I met six-year old Daniel who had leukemia, and his family. Despite their collective circumstance, Daniel's mother still had energy to feel compassion for all of the other children who had not survived. "Every night, I light candles for the memory of each child who has passed away from cancer," she told me.

How are these parents able to cope with the gravity of these circumstances? How can one even grasp that your own child is terminally ill? Where do you find the strength? It all seems so deeply....unfair. The children's lives have only just begun. I was just ranting about something pointless on Facebook while this family was praying:

a) somewhere on this planet there is a person who will donate stem cells

b) these cells are compatible with Daniel's stem cells

c) of all the children in the world, Daniel will be the lucky one who gets them

I felt pretty ridiculous and small.

I also met Anna, who has an extremely rare, untreatable, and catastrophic epilepsy syndrome. Every day, when Anna has a seizure, the family fears she will die before nursing staff can make it to where she is. The child has to be supervised 24/7—she cannot be left alone. This means the family has to put their lives to the side, stay up at night, install security cameras, and constantly worry about their child.

The strength and love these families all had in common astonished me. I have never seen such strength and perseverance as I do in them. My own illness seemed insignificant compared to them. After all, I am an adult. During filming the show I realized, for the first time in my life, how important blood and stem cell donation is. A little child's life may depend on it. Nothing is more important than paying attention to this—helping sick children. All insignificant issues and problems seemed so small and useless that I felt ashamed. And enraged.

I was in the right place, with the right people. People with tragedies greater than a failed night at a club or a bad hair day.

I was starting to find My People.

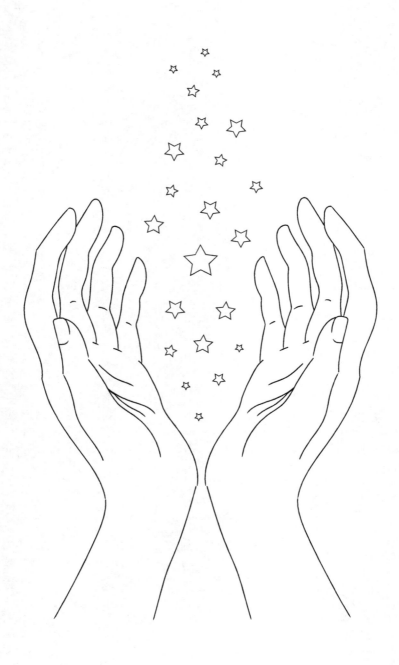

SEIZURES BEGIN

I sat on the couch with Rene, reading a story aloud. All of a sudden, my right arm started jerking up and down in a big movement. "What is going on?" I yelled. Rene looked up in terror. I tried to grab hold of my arm and stop the motion, but I could never have summoned enough strength to control it. My arm had a power all its own, power beyond my ability to control it. I screamed for Rene to quickly run next door and ask our neighbors to call an ambulance.

Rene had a quizzical look on his face at first—wondering if I was really serious—but once he saw the look of horror on my face, he realized I was not kidding, and went looking for help. At the same time, I dragged myself toward our foyer and to the front door. If Rene is unable to find our neighbors, at least someone walking their dog might see me in our front yard. My body begins convulsing in the foyer. I see our neighbors, Aki and Kirsi, running towards our house. Kirsi has her phone out and the last words I hear her yell on the phone are: "Please hurry! She's not even breathing anymore!"

I think now about my children's traumatic experience of that first seizure. I cannot even imagine the distress. Young, and alone in the house without any concept of what's happening. Will mommy die?

I'm taken to the Tampere University Hospital in an ambulance. I ask for a head MRI. My intuition itched, whispering something more than epilepsy was at work here. I had a moment of terror, and asked if it's possible the tumor has started growing again.

"That's not really how tumors work. Your tumor was just removed in an operation. It's not possible for it to reappear in a few months," my doctor told me, in slight amusement. "The seizure was probably caused by swelling in the brain, a brain edema, which was caused by the radiotherapy that you just underwent."

Life continued, but the fear remained. Yet, what could I do? Nothing could be done except hope this would be the first and last epileptic seizure of my life. What if the next seizure happens when I am taking the dogs for a walk, all on my own? I had only recently gotten up to walking all the way to the nearby forest. Now I was forced to limit my walks to set routes. If I had a seizure, someone would find me at some point. I felt limits closing in on me, and deeply sad.

I was never alone. My parents came to visit every day. They

brought food, did laundry, cleaned, and went for walks with me so I was not alone. It was in some way therapeutic to my parents accompanying me with these activities. My parents felt like there was something practical they could do, since they couldn't help me with the illness directly — this way they could be a part of it too and make a difference. When my friends found time to call, my heart would sing. Hanna came over for a coffee, Sirpa took me for a walk, Katja picked me up for a drive. I knew they all had their own, hectic lives, but they came over anyway. Everyone looked after me to make sure nothing bad happened.

Jussi took care of our family's daily life. He cooked, did the laundry, and drove the children to school and their hobbies. He learned to make green smoothies. Jussi has both peace and strength, the exact right energy I needed. The last thing I wanted were looks of pity and overly positive comments. I wanted to be around folks who listen rather than speak. I started paying attention to *how* people were talking to me.

When you are sick, even small and well-intentioned things can be annoying. "If anyone is going to make it, it'll be you." No, I did not want anyone to outdo me in my positivity. I wanted to be the one setting the pace. I will determine how positively we can think about all of this. I am *certainly not ready* to hear how someone's distant relative died of a brain tumor within a couple of months. "Call me if you need anything," is a common one. Give me a break. As if I would call busy people in the morning, asking them to cook my family a casserole, and come over and bring it to us.

What To Say (and What Not To Say) To a Sick Person:

1. *Listen.* You do not need the right words. You can just hug the person, say "Hey, I'm right here for you," and listen. *Do not give them any advice.* Only give advice if you are specifically asked to do so.

2. Do not, under any circumstances, tell horror stories of someone you knew who in a short few months died of the same disease that the person you are talking to has. No—we do not want to hear these stories.

3. Do not say, "Call me if you need anything." The sick person knows how hectic and busy other people's lives are. We will not call you during your work day. Instead, say: "Is it okay if I bring you some Indian food in the evening? Or make some macaroni casserole for your kids that you can freeze for later? Maybe take your dogs for a walk in the morning? Can I pick your kids up for a sleepover tomorrow? Hey, I'm having coffee in the city center now, would you like me to grab you a green smoothie and raw veg-

an cake before I leave?" In other words, you should give concrete suggestions. Maybe you know what your friend likes or might want. If you do not, go back to item number one: listen. We do not want to cause you any stress or ask you for anything. *We want to be able to manage on our own.* But if you really want to help us—we accept it with great gratitude. We will also never forget it. We understand if you have been unable or afraid to call us. We understand it is easier to not call us than to call us and burst into tears. We understand you wanted to see us but did not. We understand. **We are World Champions of Understanding.**

4. Do not downplay the disease. In my case, I had a very aggressive and malignant tumor. Do not say "You'll get through it." You cannot know that for sure. Do not say things you are not sure are true.

5. We want to talk about everyday things, not just our illness. You do not have to fear or underestimate your problems under the pretense that your problems are so much smaller or that they are *nothing* compared to our terminal illness. Do not hesitate to tell us if you have a cold, your child has had a vicious cycle of ear infections, you are tired, or your mar-

riage sucks. That is part of life, too. However, there is a clear difference between having something you genuinely want to talk about, and simply whining and moaning about everything, all the time. And when someone is actually very sick, they may not want to hear that you are having a bad hair day. Oh really? I lost all my hair in chemo.

6. The best thing to do is for you to come over. We can make some tea and have a talk. Nothing special, no pressure. We can talk about whatever comes up.

One night while staying in a hotel in another city, I start feeling strange. There's a feeling of confusion which slowly twists into fear. My heart starts beating fast and I panic. Help me— will it happen again? An epileptic seizure. I am all alone in a hotel room. My quick panic reaction is to run out the door. Hurry, hurry, hurry. In a state of panic, I leave all my things in my hotel room, including my wallet and phone. The door is left open, swinging on its hinges.

I run to the reception desk. There's a huge line. I cut the line past everyone as quickly as I can and yell, "I am about to have a horrible epileptic seizure, please call an ambulance immediately!" People look terrified. They give me space and don't come touch me, or ask questions.

Someone takes me to a couch in the hotel lobby, speaking

to me gently. I'm not really sure where I am anymore. The hotel manager arrives and tries to calm me down. "Everything is fine, the ambulance is coming." I tell her what is about to happen. "It's going to start soon and I'm going to lose consciousness. I need a shot from the paramedics as soon as possible."

I wake up to someone asking me the same deluge of questions that had been asked the previous time: *Do you know where you are* (no), *What is your name* (Karita) *Can you remember what happened* (no).

I'm taken to the hospital. I am not sure what kind of drugs they give me, but I wake up truly confused. I don't know who I am, what my husband's name is, where he works, where I am. I don't know if it's day or night. The room, or rather a big hall, is absolutely full of people. There is only a slight curtain separating me from the others, and I hear moaning, vomiting, and other unspecified noises from both sides of my bed. No nurses appear to be anywhere close by. I lay on a narrow bed paralyzed until I start having another seizure. "Please, someone, come over here, quickly!" I yell as loudly as I can. The panic starts rising again and my heart feels as though it will run from my chest. Two nurses come over and one of them, a young man, grabs hold of my legs. I scream *"Let go of me, don't hold onto me"* and fight back. I quickly lose consciousness and wake up even more confused than before. I have no sense of time. I have no idea what is going on. I'm packed full of drugs, I'm so confused. I don't even know if it's day or night.

I don't know how long I have been in the hospital. Should I call someone? My phone is in my hotel room. Eventually, I am able to remember my husband's name and where he works.

In the morning, I take off my pink hospital gown and ask the nurses where my jeans are. "They're here, in a plastic bag, wet...you wet yourself, ma'am-" "I'm sorry, what? What did you just say? This can't be happening. What sort of bullshit is this?!"

So there I stand, in my elegant pink hospital gown, waiting like a prom date at the hospital door and jump into Jussi's car as soon as it pulls up. We stop at the hotel to pick up my things. I mean, I do not *personally* pick them up! I sit in the car wearing my glamorous hospital gown. We take off towards Tampere, home.

More worry, more stress—and the constant fear of new seizures. My parents start spending a lot of time at our place. They bring food, do laundry, clean the house. They do not let me go for walks on my own. One morning I'm making coffee and my father sits at the table, reading the local newspaper. In passing, he asks me: "How are you doing?" I can't remember the last time someone asked me that question. I break down. I grab hold of the side of the kitchen sink to keep from collapsing. All I can say is "badly" before I dissolve into tears. My father rises to embrace me while I weep.

The truth felt too embarrassing to say out loud. I had already been asking Jussi to write my emails for me for weeks. My right hand no longer worked. Walking had also become more difficult. My right leg was not working normally. I call my doctor and beg her to let me have an MRI. She books me an urgent appointment.

I feel certain that the tumor has returned.

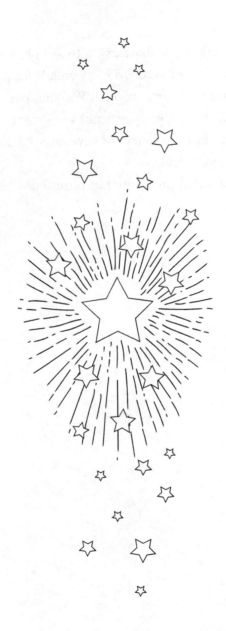

THE RETURN OF MY NOT-SO-NEW FRIEND

The doctor tells me what I already know. Everything I'm still recovering from will start again, from zero.

How many months of life have I got left? I know each surgery poses a major risk. A second operation involves greater risk than the first. I had the first operation in April, and the second would be in September. How could it have returned only a few months after surgery?

I can see only black. Emptiness. Nothingness. Darkness.

I'm aware of the limits to my strength. How are we going to break this to everyone now? Just as friends and family had overcome the shock of the first episode and started believing things might be okay. We believed it might be okay, too. All of that hell will now begin again.

In the car, on our way home from the hospital, we noted all we could do now was take things one moment at a time. The time before my second surgery was a truly dark period for me and I struggle to remember everything that went on. I cannot analyze the things I did. Every day was survival.

That was, however, something I had become practiced at.

As children, we had a lot of freedom. There were no cell phones. We were free to run around with friends outside until late in the evening. At the same time, my mother was very caring. During school skiing trips, I was always the one with the best packed lunch, home-made by Mom. People still remind me of how all my cucumber slices were cut perfectly identical, my lunch was immaculate all the way down to my bottle of juice. My family was also extremely hospitable. Friends were always welcome in my house. We had food for everyone, every person was looked after. My parents knew my friends and their parents. There was a wide safety net. My family also vacationed abroad every year in the Canary Islands. We thoroughly explored the islands on our numerous visits there. I always felt privileged my family could afford all this. Traveling was not something every child got to experience, especially in the 1980s. Even as a child, I loved to travel and I continue to love it today.

My mother worked at a tax office and my father was an entrepreneur. As children, we got used to having a full-time nanny. Our first nanny was named Pirkko. We all grew to love her very much. When she graduated from high school, the party was held in our home. Pirkko took care of us for five years. We lived in a terraced house with studio apartments upstairs, which was where all our nannies lived. We were heartbroken whenever a nanny left us. We got so attached to each one of them and remember every one of them with great warmth. Pirkko was the most caring of them all. Tarja was a great adventurer, and we always did the most exciting things with her. Marja made the best fruit custard in the world. We always had someone looking after us. We were probably in our teens when we learned to peel our own potatoes. We are still in touch with many of our former nannies and they have become our life-long friends.

My friends, or our "old gang," also supported me through many things in life. In the first grade, there were only 12 pupils in our class. I had already known some of them since kindergarten and a few more joined us along the way. We became a team. We have been through it all together: collecting stickers, going to a public swimming pool, putting on make-up for the first time in fifth grade, getting our hair permed, getting drunk for the first time and so on. All of this we did together. This bunch became my second family. We still spend a lot of time togeth- er now. We go out to eat and take trips together. It is truly unbelievable we have known each other for almost 40 years. Those years have seen all kinds of adventures, joy, and sadness.

I am sure my parents did not have it easy with me. Even though I was fairly quiet as a little girl, at the same time I was very brave and often got a talking to from a teacher or put in detention after school. The causes for this included cheating on an exam, skipping classes, and refusal to eat school lunch. We were extremely brave in doing pretty much whatever we wanted. We did artistic gymnastics, and once decided that we wanted to spend the night lying among the foam cubes in a gymnastic foam pit. We told our parents we were spend- ing the night in each other's homes. Mari at my place, me at Mari's, Noora at Suvi's place and Suvi at Noora's. Of course, our parents believed all this. After our gymnastics practice, we stayed hiding in the locker room. We packed snacks in our bags, and after everyone had left home, we sneaked into the foam pit in the gymnastics hall. We were terrified when a guard came over to make rounds during the night. They had heard some strange sounds in the hall and were already walk- ing from the door inside the hall. We held our breaths and were certain we were going to get caught. But no. We spent the whole night there, giggling away. I don't think very many people have spent the night at the Ratina gymnastics hall. But this was just so like us. We enjoyed life to the fullest.

Before the second operation, my friend Titta and I take a forest walk together. Suddenly, a dove flies right in front of us, to alight on a branch in a nearby tree. It looks straight at me, still and fragile and serene. I go home and Google the symbolic meaning of doves. The words "a new life" appear on the screen.

Unbelievable! I am sure this is a sign from somewhere above, from the Universe, from God, from something bigger. It does not matter in whom or what one believes. It is not my time to go yet. I get a tremendous amount of strength from this experience, and feel a warm sense of protection, as if I am surrounded by a large group of angels.

They have always been there, dancing and flying by my side.

Ever since I was a little girl, I have simply felt that there was always someone with me to look after me and protect me. I have felt that there is a guardian

angel beside me. Once, when I was at a confirma-
tion camp, our priest pulled me aside. They said they
saw something different in me. "You are not like the
others, do you realize that?" I still do not know what
they meant by that.

When I was studying communications at the
Paasikivi-Opisto college, one of our teachers had
cancer. He invited us for a visit at his home. We all
knew this would be our final encounter here on earth
together. We drove to his place, and as I stepped out
of the car, the moving car tire ran over my foot. I did
not dare to tell anyone what had happened. I was
not in any pain. I felt the energy of angels. I felt they
were there to protect my teacher. Soon after the vis-
it, we heard our teacher had passed away. I knew he
was in a better place.

"I have to go over the risks of the surgery with you," my surgeon says. He informs me there is a relatively large risk for
paralysis this time around. I listen to him and, in a fit of emotion blurt out: "I don't care, scrape out as much as you need
to!" Even paralysis seemed like a minor thing if that was the
cost of my life. They could do whatever they needed to. I only
wanted to live!

Again, I keep my eyes closed until I reach the operating room. They start with the preparations, again, and put the anesthetic mask over my face. "I'm counting down from ten and you will fall asleep.

10...

9...

8...

7...

....."

Beep, beep, beep, beep. My ears pick up the familiar sounds of the machines. I know I'm in the intensive care unit. I open my eyes. It's like coming back from the "other side." I'm alive! Thank God! I try to wiggle my toes, they move. Fingers. They do too. Who am I? I know who. I know where I am. Thank you! Thank you! Thank you!

Again, I first ask them to let Jussi see me at the ICU. Jussi arrives almost at the same time as my surgeon. This particular group of professionals is not exactly known for being the most sociable bunch or willing to engage in small talk with you over this and that. Nope. Surgeons think with a surgeon's brain. Theirs is a purely no-nonsense approach. That's it.

Out came a sentence that made my whole world stop: "I'm afraid it appears the tumor has become more malignant, and is now Glioblastoma Multiforme grade IV." Jussi and I look at each other. We do not say a word. Even the surgeon falls silent.

Grade IV—Glioblastoma (GBM)

Glioblastoma multiforme (GBM) is the most common and deadliest of malignant primary brain tumors in adults and is one of a group of tumors referred to as gliomas.

Mortality from the disease is 65% during the first year or observation, 90% by the end of the second year and 95% after the third year.

The standard treatment is surgery, followed by radiation therapy or combined radiation therapy and chemotherapy. If inoperable, then radiation, or radiation and chemotherapy can be administered.

The treatment requires effective teamwork from neurosurgeons, neuro-oncologists, radiation oncologists, physician's assistants, social workers, psychologists, and nurses. A supportive family environment is also helpful.

The National Center for Biotechnology Information / Focus Oncologiaie

On the second day at the hospital, I go back to ward 4 A. This time, I enjoy my time there less. This time, things are serious.

At least I no longer have to worry about the tumor becoming *more* malignant, I guess. There's no Grade five. We can't go down from here. We can only go up. Down from here is death.

This was the beginning of a new era for me. This surgery was different from the first one. It woke me up. I actually woke up. I woke up to a feeling that it was time for a *change*. While I did not know what this would mean exactly, I knew for certain that nothing could stay the same. I felt the tickle of the realization:

Everything would have to change now.

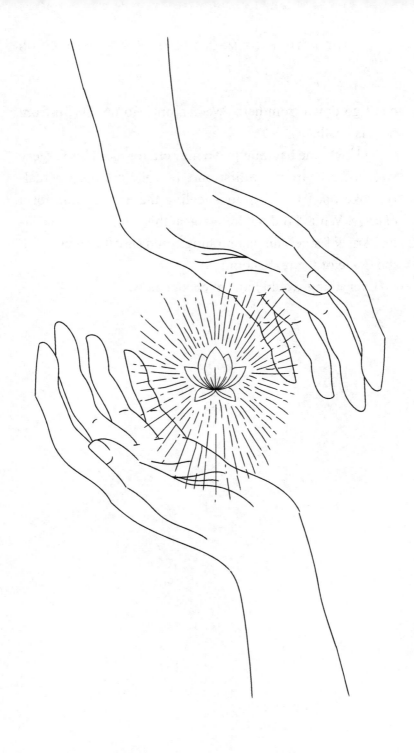

A NEW LIFE

There is my life before the surgery, and my life after. I am no longer in a hurry to get anywhere. Anywhere at all! Nothing is more important for me now than doing everything, absolutely everything, I can to get better.

After the surgery, I meet with my oncologist. My cancer treatments continue, this time in cytostatic therapy. I knew how tough this would be on my body, which was already drained—let alone the emotional stress and strain. I know I have a long cytostatic/chemo treatment coming. I understand how the cytostatic agents will destroy my immune system. Now is the time to give my body, mind, and spirit All The Support.

It is time to take personal responsibility for my own healing process. I was so used to simply doing whatever I was told, obeying and above all, not complaining. The

Finnish way is humble and not wanting to make a fuss about oneself. Also I wanted to be nice and kind to the doctors so they would be the same back to me. I figured if I behaved in a difficult way with them, the interaction would be less nice for them too. After all, I wanted to be a person the doctors want to help, not a difficult case who keeps questioning what they say. This time, I want to be involved in the decisions concerning my care and included in the process. To quote the great disability activist, James Charlton, "Nothing about us without us." No more decisions about me made without me.

When I was in the hospital, I realized I needed to find a peer-support person. I made a short list of qualities:

1. A like-minded person
2. young person
3. with the same form of tumor
4. who has a strong desire and intention to heal, no matter how bad their situation

This proved to be too tall an order, even scaling back my criteria list. The last point was the most challenging. Didn't *anyone* consider themselves capable of recovery?

"Karita, you're going to have to be that person for yourself," my nurse, Anne, said. I could've been devastated by this. I could've felt lost and alone and scared. Instead I felt empowered and strong. I will be the example I want and need. Self-supportive.

At the hospital, they gave me brochures by the local Cancer Association. *Brochures.* I remember picking them up gingerly between my fingers, as one would pick up some cat vomit, walking to the nearest trash can, and dropping them in. This was the starting point for rebuilding my life from scratch.

I begin a massive information search, while still not Googling my diagnosis. Keyword searches: healing cancer, healing diet, diet and cancer, alternative therapies, cancer survivors.

It was as if I had entered a different world. I felt all my old interests taking a back seat and becoming replaced by something new that was endlessly fascinating and interesting to me. It felt empowering, these are the people I want to be with and the subject matter I want to be with. This is my source of support—support which I can't get from the side of the medicine and science, the doctor's side of things.

Entering spirituality felt like lights going off inside my mind and awaking to something new. It energized me. Hope started trickling in more and more.

There's so much that we can't explain with logic and reason alone. That world started opening up to me.

I read studies about how cancer is treated in other countries. For instance, how complementary therapies are used alongside medicine in Germany. In Switzerland, complementary therapies, such as anthroposophical medicine, classic homeopathy, traditional Chinese medicine and herbal medicine are accepted as forms of treatment supporting the official cancer treatments. Here in Finland, around one third of adults also use complementary treatments in support of the medical care they receive. I read about different forms of treatment, from the CyberKnife radiosurgery device to the use of medical marijuana. My reflexologist, Kirsi Sarimaa, also awakens me to the harm caused by dental bacteria and amalgam fillings (which are now banned in Finland due to the aluminum absorbing into the blood stream), and makes me understand more about the importance of oral, dental and gum wellness. The mucous membranes of the mouth serve as a pathway for bacteria to enter the bloodstream.

Little by little, I start forming a small group with other people experiencing brain tumors. As our group grows larger, we are able to form our peer group under the local cancer society, and we start holding our meetings there. Getting to talk with other people who have been through the same things gave us all a feeling of support and connection—two vital aspects of human need.

I still sometimes go there today. Esa and I are the only original members still in the group. All the other founding members have died. Needless to say, it is not uncommon to hear bad news in our group.

I flip my mindset and start perceiving the cytostatic drugs not as something toxic but rather as a therapeutic substances. I imagine them as chemical secret agents, treating my condition. I imagine the agents sneaking to my head, making the remaining cancer cells "heal" or die down. I do a lot of mental practices in connection with the cytostatic therapy. I do not want to picture all these horrible toxic agents filling my body, fighting inside of me. I am not interested in fighting anything. That would be the same as thinking something "bad" is inside me. No!! That thought does not take me anywhere. Instead, I treat the tumor with all the love that I have inside of me. My not-so-new friend came to make me slow my pace and teach me boundaries. **This tumor is a friend that has come here to help me, to teach me to live a life better aligned with my personal values.**

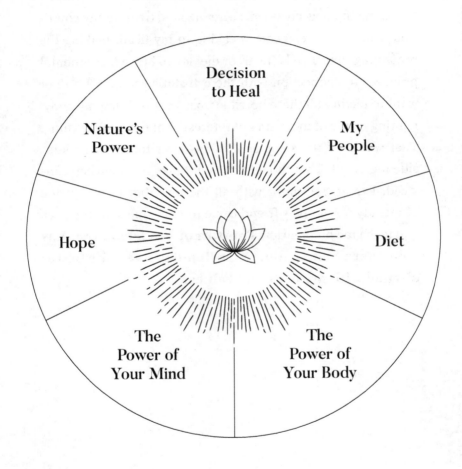

THE HEALING CIRCLE

I refuse to give up. Nope. I want to live! I knew I would need all the strength I could gather. I formed a Healing Circle comprised of seven different areas:

1) The Decision to Heal
2) My People
3) Diet
4) The Power of the Body
5) The Power of the Mind
6) The Importance of Hope for Healing
7) The Power of Nature

The Decision to Heal

I decide if no one has ever healed from my condition before, someone would have to be the first. I focus my thoughts on reasons for living—not reasons why I do not want to die. I truly want to live. I love life. I have two of the most amazing children in the world, and they genuinely need me. I am full of dreams. There are still so many countries I want to visit and explore. So many things I want.

To see and experience things.

To laugh with my friends with tears in my eyes.

To see my boys grow up, their confirmation parties, their weddings.

I want to be a grandmother someday.

I write the word "impossible" on a piece of paper and cross out two choice letters.

I decide to do everything I can for my recovery. This means putting work aside without hesitation, handing my hosting gigs over to others. From now on, my mission: working on my own healing and clearly setting my focus on healing—not on my illness. There is a strong difference between framing one's life in terms of wellness or illness. I will let you, gentle reader, consider it yourself.

My People

I decide I will only surround myself with people who *sincerely believe* I can heal. Lo and behold, the right people just start showing up in front of me. This may seem familiar to you: you are sitting somewhere, let's say in a café, and just happen to start chatting with the person standing in front of you in the line to the counter. And it turns out that the person happens to be a reflexologist or an acupuncturist. I had innumerable encounters like that. It is the law of attraction—you get what you are looking for.

In psychology, they talk about frequency bias, or Baader-Meinhof Phenomenon—when you notice something once, and then it begins to turn up everywhere. Maybe it was there all the time, you just never noticed. Maybe it's as simple as coincidence. Or maybe sometimes our inner thoughts line up with that which occurs outside. Maybe the inside lines up with the outside. I choose to believe that means I'm on the right track.

I found it extremely important to include a medical specialist among my people. I had read several books by Antti Heikkilä, and admired his courage to publicly state his opinions which were often contrary to the mainstream view, in connection with the food pyramid, for instance. I admire his courage to resist conforming to the majority.

I book an appointment with him at the Eira Hospital in Helsinki. I am not sure what kind of help I expect to get from him, but I know he has a lot of knowledge about the importance of nutrition for healing. Our meeting has a warm atmosphere. Antti opens by saying: "I know we'll figure out something, Karita."

These are the first words of hope anyone has given me

throughout the entire ordeal. Yes, this far in. It was like taking a cool shower on a very hot day, such relief hearing a medical professional offer some kind of confidence in recovery. Never underestimate the power of simple encouragement, especially if you are in a role as an expert or authority.

Another person I counted as part of My People was Elina, who worked at the Ruohonjuuri health food store. "Hey, I know someone you have to meet," she said. I trust her completely, and agree to meet John, a reiki practitioner. The first thing he says to me is, "I can see you talk for a living, but you spend your time talking about all the wrong things." Wait, how could John know what I did for a living?! Just a few days previously I had the thought that I wanted to—or rather that I should—spend my time talking about something significant. Something that actually mattered.

At the time, my hosting gigs more or less involved events taking place at malls, going on about some promotion or other. Even though I enjoyed (and still enjoy) these gigs, they usually involve an excessive "Buy this, buy that...look how inexpensive that is!" type of overexcited chit-chat. At times, I also had to promote products I personally did not believe in or which I would never actually personally use. And here I was, in front of a complete stranger, who could see all of this in me before I had even spoken a word to him.

"Your purpose here is to talk about something meaningful and important, you know?" Well, I did know that - and at the same time I did not. I mean, I knew that I should, but *what* exactly should I be talking about?

But that was not the point of our meeting.

John outlines essential oils which can support our health and will help my body find balance. He recommends an essential oil for me: frankincense. I have never heard anything about it, but I hear the voice of intuition going off inside of me: "Yes, yes, yes!"

Essential oils are aromatic volatile compounds derived from natural sources, such as bushes, trees, flowers, roots and seeds. They are typically extracted by steam distillation, water distillation or cold press. Essential oils play many roles and have different characteristics in plants. Essential oils contain oxygen molecules, which help transporting nutrients around plants to the cells that require these. As the lack of nutrients often leads to a lack of oxygen, diseases (e.g. various fungal diseases, bacterial diseases, and viruses) start to emerge as cells lack essential nutrients and oxygen.

As essential oils provide cells with the oxygen that is vital to them, they simultaneously stimulate the immune system. Essential oils also have characteristics that promote healing. In plants, essential oils also serve as a defense mechanism against external threats and damage.

The strength of essential oils lies in the synergies of their components (the cumulative effect of two or more contributing factors). Each essential oil includes between 200 and 500 different bioingredients, as a result of which the oils have versatile effects. No two oils are the same.

Essential oils have a unique, fat-soluble structure, which is highly similar with our cellular structure. The molecules that make up essential oils are relatively small, which increases their capacity to penetrate cell membranes in the human body.

The therapeutic effects of essential oils depend fully on the quality of the oil, its organic chemical ingredients and their interrelationships. As a result, it is extremely important to have thorough knowledge of the background of any essential oil you are using: where it comes from, how it is produced, which quality standards apply to it, and for which purposes can it be used.

Pure essential oils intended for therapeutic purposes have effects that support wellbeing, and they are effective for uses such as maintaining normal hormone functions and immunity, hair care and skincare, and supporting overall well being.

Pure essential oils intended for therapeutic purposes will reach each cell of the human body in around 20 minutes, after which the oil is metabolized, or broken down, by the human metabolism.

(Reference: Essential Oils Desk Reference, Life Science Publishing 2019)

We also discuss diet. I tell John that while I am a vegetarian, I have not really found "the right one," a diet that perfectly suits me, one which would both help my healing process and appeal to my senses. John promises to travel to Tampere (all for me!) to give a macrobiotic food course so that I can learn more. Agreed!

Others I counted as My People included my nearest and dearest: my own family, my parents, my sisters, friends, and relatives. What all these individuals had in common was their sincere desire to help me, a belief in the possibility of healing, and an amazing drive—something they all had in abundance. None of these people were lamenting, regretting or pitying my circumstances, going "Oh, what terrible luck you have!" No. These were people who could simply act, and were full of energy, faith, strength, and perseverance.

There was also one more group that became part of My People: everyone whose lives had been touched by cancer.

Diet

Diet is a topic that never fails to invoke reactions. What is right and what is wrong? What should I really eat to stay healthy or heal? Does diet matter?

In my old life, before cancer, my diet was primarily composed of yogurt and bread. Some yogurt and bread for breakfast, and coffee with milk to drink. Whatever I could get my hands on for lunch, which often meant more yogurt and bread. Some coffee in the afternoon and maybe a warm meal in the evening. A piece of bread for a late-night snack. I took my health for granted, and thought nothing more of it. I always thought of myself as a healthy person.

But was I, really? When I was a child, they should have given me a VIP pass at the dentist's. I ate ridiculous amounts of candy and ice cream, drank cola and consumed anything sweet I could get my hands on. There were always cavities in my teeth. As I grew older, I spent little time thinking about food. I thought I had a healthy lifestyle. After all, I ate vegetarian meals, exercised, and did yoga. I read spiritual literature such as Wayne Dyer, Paul Coelho, yoga books, Ayurveda, Chinese medicine, mind-body-spirit books, and anything having to do with spiritual health.

I have tried keeping this section on diet simple and comprehensible, without going into too many details or relying too much on research. I want to emphasize here that I am neither a doctor nor a dietitian. **Everything I have written in this section is based on my personal choices that have felt right to me based on my experience, intuition, and independent study.**

I consider it extremely important to point out here there is no single diet universally right for everyone. Instead, everyone should do their research, both anecdotally and scientifically. If something in this section resonates with you and calls out your name, try it for yourself.

In countries such as Denmark, the United States, India and Germany, diet plays a far greater role in cancer treatment than it does here in Finland. In fact, the unfortunate thing is that diet plays *no* role in Finnish cancer care. "Eat whatever feels right," "the main thing is that you are eating," "it really doesn't matter what you eat, it has *no effect* on your healing." So many times, I have heard such phrases from doctors. I understand that they are not experts in nutrition. My job, as far as they are concerned, is just to rely on their expertise in medicine. The level of medicine is great here in Finland and something we can be very satisfied with. There are not enough words to describe how thankful I am for Timo Tähtinen, the brain surgeon who operated on me twice. I am extremely thankful to the intensive care unit, radiotherapy nurses, and my wonderful cancer specialists at the Tampere University Hospital. I know they would do everything in their power to help their patients.

That being said, my greatest mission is to illustrate how Western medicine and complementary treatments can go hand-in-hand during cancer treatment. Instead of pitting these forms of therapy against each other, they should *support* each other.

You should also note I have intentionally chosen to use the term *complementary* therapies—not alternative therapies. This is as I feel that using the word "alternative" would suggest only one form of therapy may be used. That would mean either accepting medical treatment or going full hippie and trying to find a cure with "natural" methods. Instead, I feel neither of these treatment forms should cancel out the other. As it so happens, the purpose of complementary therapies is to *complement* medical treatment. What a shock, wonder why they would call it complementary then, hmmmmm...

I also refuse to take a stand on what therapies people should choose. For example, if someone is unwilling to undergo cytostatic therapy, and opts for natural methods instead, that is that individual's personal decision to make. Similarly, if a person wants to be subjected to every medical treatment there is and does not believe in the effectiveness of any other form of therapy, so be it.

Personally, I have chosen to use both treatment forms. I believe in Western medicine and I believe in complementary therapies, and I have strong faith in diet as well. My intuition said a big "yes" to a change. I knew I had to change so many things in my life and daily routine. That included the way I thought, what I was eating and drinking, how I accomplished tasks, and what I believed in. It matters whether I am actively contributing to my healing or remain a helpless victim waiting for doctors to come and save me.

It took some time for me to find an appropriate diet, and it will probably take you time as well. Before the surgery, putting my sodium balance in order was the first thing I decided to do. Salts are vital for humans. Natrium plays a significant role in our cell metabolism. The warnings about the harmful health effects of salt concern the regular, white table salt. By contrast, sea salt contains elements vital to in regulation of bodily functions, and contain more than 90 important minerals. Our bodies need salt to work. A lack of salt will cause "interruptions" in the electric functions of the body (electrical impulses, cellular metabolism, etc). I use both sea salt and Himalayan salt.

Each cell in the human body needs the right kinds of building materials, known as nutrients, to keep its health and create new, functional cells. I started taking vitamins and minerals, and drinking vitamin and antioxidant beverages. I found the most helpful supplements to be:

- Vitamin B that has all B vitamins, C, D3
- selenium
- magnesium
- Q10

- matcha / sencha green tea
- turmeric, ginger, spirulina, chlorella, wheatgrass, reishi, chaga

I also started making green smoothies and my own juices. After participating in a macrobiotic course by John, the Reiki instructor, I knew I had found my way home. This was it—this was my diet. Macrobiotic diet aims at achieving physical and mental well-being through food that promotes finding energetic balance. This is typically a very well-balanced diet that includes a lot of fibers, good fats, a lot of vegetables and seeds, vegetable protein, and a limited amount of meat. It also puts emphasis on organic and varied food.

I found it important not to pay too much attention to details. It simply does not seem right to me to follow a diet religiously or "orthodoxically." I don't believe in the myth of Purity—there is no such thing! Macrobiotic diet has many good things going for it. But it should not cause you any stress. For instance, I love coffee, so I never gave it up. (I *did* change to an organic variety).

It is important to understand the liver plays an extremely important role in health, especially in the treatment of illnesses. The liver clears our blood of toxins accumulating in our bodies as a result of a poor diet and beverages, alcohol, and coffee—and let's not even talk about additives and environmental toxins. We can help the liver by eating food as pure and nutrient-rich as possible. Excessive amounts of sugar and poor fats disturb liver functions. The liver also eliminates cancer cells, which all of us (including healthy people) have in our bodies. Indeed, paying attention to liver health and functions before, during, and after cancer treatments is essential.

The food we eat should primarily be plant-based and consist of fresh green leafy vegetables, natural herbs, berries, fruit, different vegetables, good fats, nuts, and seeds. A diet rich in these ingredients provides us with enough antioxidants, protective nutrients, vitamins, enzymes, minerals, fibers, and all the carbohydrates we need.

A healthy and varied diet affects our brain through the intestine. The intestine affects the immune system and hormone production. Failure to absorb nutrients interrupts cell regeneration and restoration, energy production, immunity, and helpful bacteria.

I wish nutrition was better utilized in the treatment of cancer as well as other diseases—also as part of the official guidelines. Having to do all the work for yourself to find the right information did not seem right to me. Nothing was available and ready. Diet is simply not discussed in Finnish cancer care. Or, if the topic is addressed, the discussion revolves around the food pyramid, which is used as the basis of nutrition in Finnish health care. It includes a lot of bread, margarine, and milk.

Grocery stores are filled with industrially-produced food, mass-manufactured from poor-quality ingredients. There are a lot of "fat-free" or low-fat products on the market, where fats have been replaced with a massive amount of sugar. I started reading the product descriptions of items sold in grocery stores. If a description was filled with serial codes and E numbers, I put the product back on the shelf. Prepackaged food, also known as convenience food, usually contains a large number of additives, coloring, and preservatives. These are added to food products to preserve the freshness of the product for longer and make its color and appearance as appealing to buyers as possible. While these additives are approved by the USDA and FDA, it does not mean these components are harmless, let alone healthy. We cannot be certain about the combined effects of different E-numbered components.

Because of all this, I have made a choice to select foods and beverages as close to their natural form as possible whenever I am grocery shopping. I also try and choose food that is as locally produced as possible, for ecological reasons. I eliminated all store-bought juices and any sugary or synthetic sugar drinks from my diet and replaced them with plenty of water. Even an old Finnish proverb knows it: "Water is the oldest medicine." It would be best to collect water straight from a natural spring, which there are plenty of here in Finland. Water is the basis for all health, as it flushes toxins from the body. Tap water often contains chlorine, fluoride and heavy metals, all of which have been found to cause cancer. It would be best to purchase a filtering system for the home that removes harmful agents from the tap water. Sometimes, when I am driving home from a gig in Helsinki, I pop by to a natural water spring located on the way in Lempäälä to collect spring water. I can honestly say that the water from the spring tastes much cleaner and better than any other water. But the fact is, I often do not have the time. Or the energy. I also drink water from the tap or use a filter jug to purify.

A cancer prevention diet also fosters the prevention and treatment of type 2 diabetes and many other diseases. It also contributes to the maintenance of overall health. It would be a good idea to eliminate meat, dairy, processed foods, and all refined sugars from your diet. At the minimum, it is advisable to radically cut down on these products, or, if you choose to keep consuming them, at least favor organic products and ingredients that have been processed as little as possible. Baby steps!

I consider sugar particularly harmful—after all, we do not want to feed our cancer cells. Instead of refined sugar, you should make sure your diet includes a lot of berries, and organic fruit and vegetables, eat healthy non-animal based proteins contained by sources such as beans, nuts and seeds, use good fats and oils, and increase the amount of healthy herbs and spices in your diet. There's a lot of coding surrounding sugar, "brown rice syrup," "sucralose," etc. Any kind of syrup is a sugar. In the US, there is a sugar called "high-fructose corn syrup." This sugar is especially destructive because it is so heavily altered from its original form. In Finnish we have a word for it: *piilosokeri*. It translates to "hidden sugar" or "hiding sugar." Meaning, so many foods have sugar in some form, and you wouldn't even know. You might accidentally eat a lot of *piilosokeri* because you didn't realise salad dressing or pasta sauce has a ton of it, for example.

Good bacteria feeds a healthy bacterial population in your body and promotes intestinal function. We get good bacteria from fermented products, such as sauerkraut and fermented carrots. We get high-quality lactic acid bacteria from probiotic products, such as the Boris beverage available in Finland, which has been produced using traditional methods and contains live lactic cultures. It is a probiotic drink, containing organic ingredients: beets, lingonberry, cabbage, carrot, mountain salt, well-water. Kind of like Finnish kombucha!

What about milk—so popular in Finland that it is practically treated as our national beverage? The mental image of cows happily grazing on a pasture persists. Today's milk production is a world away from that. The quality of milk is reduced by the immobility and stress experienced by the animals, in addition to the antibiotics administered. This means milk is no longer as pure as it used to be, even at the moment of milking. Its nutritional value is also reduced by industrial processing. Before ending up on a shelf in a grocery store, milk is pasteurized (heated up) and homogenized (fats are broken down). What does this mean in practice, then? Heating up milk results in killing off good microbes, bacteria and enzymes, which help digestion, changing the quality of the protein and destroying most nutrients. Homogenization is mostly carried out for aesthetic reasons, to prevent the natural fat from the milk from rising up to its surface. However, doing this also results in eliminating the fats that are very good for us.

While we can also get calcium from vegetables, the need for calcium supplements varies from one person to the next. The best non-animal origin sources of calcium include leafy greens, such as broccoli, kale, nettle, and sesame seeds, almonds, dried figs, and other nuts and seeds.

I limit my dairy intake to milk in my coffee, and might add a few spoonfuls of Greek, unflavored organic yogurt to my breakfast consisting of nuts, berries and fruit. And I love cheese, eating it a few times a week. Remember. It's all about the balance!

Enjoying food without any pangs of guilty conscience or feelings of guilt is just as important. Everything in moderation.

Have you ever thought about why bread is so addictive? You always need more of it. One slice is rarely enough. Bread is a typical example of a processed food. Wheat has been processed from its original seed form by purification and milling it into fine flour, and then sugar and salt are added. After this, the bread is sold in a plastic bag to maximize its shelf life. A bread like this has an extremely high glycemic index which means the carbohydrates quickly convert into glucose or, simply put, sugar, used by the cells. And we know by now that cancer cells love sugar. And boy, oh boy, is that sugar addictive. Because of all this, it is a good idea to eliminate white flour from your diet altogether and replace it with higher quality alternatives, such as millet and buckwheat.

Good fats safeguard the absorption of antioxidants and feed the brain and all cells in the body. Our bodies depend on high-quality fats. This is a considerably controversial topic that never fails to provoke discussion and a variety of opinions. The fats in my diet come from avocados, nuts, fish, organic eggs, olive oil and organic butter, and high-quality omega 3 cod liver oil.

In Finland, we use a lot of margarine. The history of margarine is pretty interesting: a French chemist invented it in the late 1800s as an inexpensive butter substitute. It was intended for military and lower class use. In the 1980s, it became popular as an unsaturated fat alternative to butter. Now of course we know that margarine is too highly processed to be considered healthy. But, it's still popular here in Finland due to a number of factors, including long shelf life and, quite simply, tradition.

I use coconut oil for frying and add a spoonful of it in my smoothies. Coconut oil is also useful as a basic lotion used for skin, suitable for the whole family. I also use organic virgin oliveoil, MCT oil, caprylic acid, primrose oil, hemp oil, and avocado oil internally.

I advise you to pay attention to the quality of the fats you use. Polyunsaturated fatty acids (omega 3 and omega 6) are known as vital fatty acids, as our bodies are incapable of producing them on their own. Getting enough omega 6 is no problem, as we tend to get plenty, even too much of it. Omega 6 is found in most vegetable oils, whole grain breads, poultry, and eggs. However, we usually get a lot less omega 3 fatty acids. Fluctuation in the balance of these fatty acids has damaging consequences, such as cardiovascular diseases and also chronic diseases, including cancer. Omega-3 fatty acids are vital for the formation of molecules that prevent infections. We therefore need omega 3 and omega 6 in a suitable proportion.

Oily fish, such as mackerel, sardine or salmon, are an important source of omega-3 fatty acids, EPA, and DHA. Omega-3 fatty acids mostly accumulate in the fish as a result of phytoplankton and zooplankton, which the fish feed on. We can easily add omega-3 fatty acids to our diet by putting ground flaxseed in porridge or smoothies, for instance. Studies have explored the effects of fish oil on children's ability to focus and learn as well as in treating ADHD, autism, and depression. It is a good idea to include fish oil in children's diet.

The industrial processing of fatty acids in their natural state, which is done in the context of different "low fat" products (including margarine and other spreads), results in trans fats, which are unnatural and may cause cell damage.

Products to avoid:
- white flour
- white sugar
- industrially produced oils and margarines
- trans fats, i.e. products containing partly or fully hydrogenated fats, such as cookies, potato chips, chocolate, candy, and sweet pastries
- industrially produced convenience foods
- foods containing additives, preservatives, coloring, corn syrup, fructose, or aspartame
- sausages, cold cuts, red meat
- industrially produced juices
- energy drinks and soft drinks
- large amounts of alcohol

Precision Products to Prevent and Treat Cancer

Cancer researchers Richard Beliveau and Denis Gingras investigated the effects of various foods on cancer in their book, *Foods That Fight Cancer*. Many food products, including spices, green tea, turmeric, lemon, and cruciferous vegetables, have proven effects on cancer cells. Studies have shown how the natural components of such foods can biochemically prevent and combat the development of cancer.

You should favor ingredients such as the following:
Cruciferous vegetables, including kale, broccoli and cauliflower, brussels sprouts
Cruciferous vegetables contain ingredients that can stop cancer cells from growing, prevent them from metastasizing, or even kill off cancer cells. Cruciferous vegetables contain a wide range of cancer-preventing biomolecules.

Garlic and onion
Garlic and onion delay the development of cancer, protect cells against damage caused by carcinogens, and prevent cancer cells from multiplying. Chewing on garlic or onion makes the plant release cancer-combating molecules. Eating onions provides the overall best way to ingest cancer-fighting molecules.

Turmeric
Turmeric is one of the most important medical agents of Ayurveda, a traditional system of medicine from India. Turmeric treats infections, digestive disorders, fever, and liver infections. It may provide one explanation to the major differences in the incidence of cancer between Asia and Western countries. Curcumin, the most important ingredient in turmeric, is a biomolecule with versatile medical effects, as it prevents blood

clots, lowers cholesterol and is an effective antioxidant (exceeding the effectiveness of vitamin E several times over) and contains cancer-fighting compounds. Good results have also been achieved with cancer cells grown in a laboratory: curcumin has been astonishingly effective in preventing the growth of cells isolated from cancerous tumors in humans. These studies have involved sort of exhausting the cancer cells, leaving the tumor without nutrients and energy, and this has resulted in the apoptosis, or cell death, of cancer cells.

Green tea
Similarly as turmeric, green tea contains an exceptionally high amount of biomolecules that effectively prevent cancer—especially macha and sencha teas. An analysis of different varieties of green tea has noted that there is major variation in the amount of epigallocatechin gallate (EGCG) released during the brewing of green tea, and Japanese green tea is generally of higher quality than Chinese. I personally aim to drink green tea every day. I always mix in some manuka honey, which has natural antibacterial properties. Mānuka honey has been found to have medicinal value and has been studied a lot since the 1960s. Thus far, the research findings have indicated that the honey is also effective in treating resistant bacteria. The honey can also help with stomach issues, intestinal illnesses, heartburn and fungal infections, and can be used in treating the same ailments as regular honey.

Lemon

Lemon contains a significant amount of flavonoids, which contribute to maintaining health. Lemon helps with the secretion of carcinogenic substances from the body. It is very easy to get vitamin C naturally by squeezing half a lemon in water every morning.

Beetroot

Beetroot contains a lot of health-promoting compounds. It is also a natural remedy for those with high blood pressure.

Chaga mushroom, reishi, and other mushrooms

These medicinal mushrooms are known to support the body's natural immunity and protect our cells from free radicals.

Wheatgrass, spirulina, and chlorella

Wheatgrass contains a variety of substances maintaining the health of the body: minerals, vitamins, amino acids, chlorophyll, and enzymes beneficial for the body. Spirulina is a great source of protein and boosts up the metabolism, removes toxins from the body, balances the bacterial strain, and contains large amounts of chlorophyll—the green pigments found in plants—which increase the alkalinity of the body. Spirulina contains a vast amount of minerals that are important to the body, including selenium, calcium and sulphate. Chlorella supports brain and liver functions, improves digestion, and helps the regeneration of bodily tissues. It reduces infections and improves the functions of the immune system. This is significant as the immune system of cancer patients is often in poor shape because of the disease as well as the use of cytostatic agents.

My Personal Food Philosophy

Over half of my diet consists of vegetables; around 60% of the food I eat is raw and 40% is cooked. I am a pescatarian, so my diet contains no meat. I do occasionally eat some fish, though. I start my mornings by squeezing lemon in tepid water. After this, I make my "witches' brew," which consists of ingredients such as turmeric and black pepper mixed with water, and a green smoothie, which typically contains wheatgrass, spirulina, chlorella, good fats like avocado or nuts, and either berries or greens. My breakfast itself often consists of a couple of tablespoons of Greek yogurt and some berries (say, blueberries, raspberries, black currants, or lingonberries). I top it all with some cocoa nibs and chia or flax seed, and pieces of fruit such as pineapple, pear or banana. Overnight oats, soaked in almond or oat milk is also a lovely way to start my day.

At some point during the day, I typically make a green smoothie or freshly squeezed juice. When I make a smoothie, I often put in kale and spinach, and, if it is summer, some edible wild plants, such as nettle, lady's mantle and daffodils, banana, pear or pineapple, avocado (for all those good fats), and nuts and seeds (for more good fats), including chia seeds, flax seeds, Brazil nuts, cashews, walnuts, coconut oil, or a sprinkle of MCT oil and water. If I do not make a smoothie, I usually make juice out of carrot, celery, turmeric, ginger and wheatgrass.

I eat plant-based meals for lunch and dinner, typically heated ones: woks, soups, salads big enough to keep me full, vegetable stews and a lot of raw foods. When you are navigating which diet is best for you, I recommend reading up on Ayurveda, the Indian system of medicine, and its three bodily humors: Vata, Pitta and Kapha. Based on the system, I belong to the Vata-Pitta category (mostly Vata, which means cold— that is why I favor warm meals as they balance the Vata). I provide a little snapshot of an Ayurvedic diet later in the book, don't worry!

Eating clean, genuine food is the main thing. Clean food means food whose production and cultivation has involved as few industrial chemicals as possible (such as pesticides, additives and coloring), and whose production processes include as little exposure to toxic agents as possible. I'm not wild about the word clean used here, as it has moral implications. But for the moment, try to define it by the terms provided.

What I Eat in a Day!

BREAKFAST:
A big glass of water with lemon.
Oats with lots of berries, nuts, and seeds and organic Greek / soy yogurt + green smoothie (or I make a fresh juice), or an omelette with spinach and tomatoes—and a generous dollop of olive oil
And coffee—of course!

LUNCH:
Oven-roasted veggies, fish + salad with good fats added to it like avocado and olive oil and nuts

DINNER:
Veggie dish with rice

FOR SNACKS:
Nuts, smoothie, fruits, berries

Green juices and smoothies

The main difference between green juices and green smoothies has to do with texture: green smoothies include fiber and juices do not. Think about what your body needs right at this moment. Smoothies fill you up more and it is easy to include good fats in them by adding ingredients such as nuts or avocados; juices are lighter and gentler to your digestion.

I think it's a good idea to make one part of your daily routine before introducing the second one. You need a juicer or juice compressor for making juice. Making juice is easier, as you can put anything you come up with in the juicer. A good rule of thumb is to use ingredients you like but do not use very often in your daily life. You should not overthink it. Just let loose, experiment and enjoy!

In the summer, it is a great idea to use wild ingredients you pick up from the wilderness. Now that's superfood at its finest!

Here are a few of my favorite smoothie, juice, and overnight oat recipes.

Karita's special juices and smoothies

ENERGY TO ENLIVEN YOU
a handful of kale
a handful of spinach
1 avocado
1 banana
1 pear
nuts
a few pieces of fresh turmeric
a sprinkle of caprylic acid or 1 tbsp coconut oil
water

GREEN POWER
daffodil leaves
spinach
1 avocado
1 chunk of pineapple
1 apple
chia seeds (add water: chia gel)
hemp seeds
flax seeds
water

SUPERMOM (by Juiceman)
400 ml almond milk or milk of your choice
1 tbsp hemp oil
1 tsp wheatgrass powder
1 tbsp flaxseeds
a dash of vanilla extract
a few mint leaves
a handful of spinach leaves
a few kale leaves
1/4 a cucumber, chopped
a few dates, pitted
1/2 an avocado, peeled and pitted
a handful of frozen strawberries
1 frozen banana

KARITA'S FRESH SUMMER JUICE
daffodil leaves
lady's mantle leaves
1 orange
a piece of cucumber
a piece of ginger
1 pear
1 lemon

MORNING BOOSTER

a few celery stalks

4 carrots

1 lemon

1/2 cucumber

NATURAL STRENGTH

daffodil leaves

nettle

1 lemon

a few celery stalks

1 apple

a few pieces of fresh turmeric

GREEN HIPPIE

nettle

daffodil

1/2 zucchini

1 apple

FALLTIME FLAIR

1 beetroot

4 carrots

1/2 sweet potato

2 pieces of fresh turmeric

MORNING GLORIOUS JUICE (by Kris Carr)

1 large cucumber

a fistful kale

a fistful romaine

3 stalks celery

1 big broccoli stem

1 green apple, quartered

½ peeled lemon, quartered

Nordic superfoods

Here in Finland, we have the best superfoods growing right under our feet. I typically eat berries as they are. (Due to our "freedom to roam" or "everyman's right," we have the right to go anywhere in nature and pick berries or mushrooms, enjoy them or even sell them, camp out, hike, or swim in any of our 168,000 lakes). Many people like to make berry smoothies, which is also an excellent way of ingesting antioxidants. The smoothies I make are mostly green ones, but I also eat berries every day, for instance in overnight oats or on their own. It does not matter in which form you choose to eat berries, the main thing is that you eat a wide variety of berries: blueberries, strawberries, raspberries, cranberries, cloudberries, blackcurrants...

Virpi Raipala-Cormier is a Finnish "guru" on edible wild

plants, herbs, and natural healing, and someone I really admire. Her life's work is exploring the healing properties of
natural herbs, and she has supported me immensely in my
journey towards healing. According to Virpi, the onset of an
illness is influenced by both karmic and genetic aspects as
well as lifestyles, mind, worries, stress, the environment, poor
diet, immobility, alcohol, and red meat.

Below are the most important herbs for strengthening your
immunity and treating cancer:

*Wheatgrass is the most important purifier of all raw foods,
strengthening your life force and improving your resistance.
It contains a huge amount of chlorophyll and a lot of vitamins
(vitamins B1, B2, B6 and C). In fact, wheatgrass juice is one of
the basics used by the Hippocrates Health Institute, a holistic
institute for cancer care. Think of wheatgrass juice as a sort
of liquid oxygen. Wheatgrass contains a lot of iron. It is also
advisable to drink wheatgrass juice after surgery, for instance,
if you are struggling with low hemoglobin. Start with a small
amount, such as a teaspoonful.

- Nettle strengthens and nurtures your blood. It contains multiple vitamins, including vitamins C, B, D
  and E as well as minerals. Nettle gives you energy,
  strength, and supports your kidneys. Your kidneys
  are the source of your body's physical and mental
  wellbeing, a resource for your health.

- Yarrow increases white blood cell activity, improves your immunologic resistance, and helps with fatigue and stress. It is a good idea to have two cups of yarrow tea before noon.

- Daffodil removes toxins from your body and is a liver remedy.

- Mushrooms and edible polypores (chaga) are commonly used for therapeutic purposes, particularly in Russia. Chaga mushroom is a major source of antioxidants.

- Flaxseeds nurture your stomach, intestine, heart, and blood vessels. They are a great source of fiber, protein, and omega-3 fatty acids. According to studies, flaxseeds help prevent the development of breast cancer. This means you should include flaxseeds in your daily diet. It is easy to sprinkle some on your oats or in a smoothie, for instance.

Dietary supplements and vitamins

My interest in holistic health was further piqued when I visited Kaarlo Jaakkola at his Antioxidant Clinic for extensive bloodwork. As my body had been clearly weakened by surgery, radiotherapy, cytostatic therapy and stress, supporting and strengthening my resistance felt like the right thing to do. This involved providing my body with the protective nutrients, vitamins, minerals and trace elements that it lacked.

Doctors emphasize that we do not know enough about the combined effect of vitamins and cytostatic drugs. I am sure that is true. This is why one should exercise caution, investigate, and consider what is the best and safest option for you. I felt that as my body was famished and weak, it needed support with certain vitamins and antioxidants.

We know supplements cannot replace the effects of natural sources (berries, vegetables, fruit). The best way to get necessary vitamins is through food—in their natural and original form. There is no wonder drug to compensate for a poor diet lacking nutrients.

The following supplements were important to me: probiotics, vitamins B12, B, D and C, Q10, arginine, alpha lipoic acid, zinc, silica (silicic acid gel), selenium, magnesium, iron, folic acid, and cod liver oil, which contains both EPA and DHA fatty acids. Gradually, once I started feeling that my body was more balanced, I reduced my use of vitamins and aimed to instead ingest them in their natural, original form, such as in vegetables, berries, pressed juices and smoothies. Baby steps!

Every person is whole and all our different parts are in constant interaction. The right kind of nutrition is also strongly connected to spiritual growth. It may be very difficult for us to make progress on our path of spiritual growth, if we keep feeding our bodies with completely inappropriate, harmful nutrition. All kinds of addictions, emotional eating, and the chemicals ingested in food can also block our body's natural flow. These blocks prevent us from reaching our inner potential.

The Power of the Body

Our bodies want to be well. They are constantly seeking a balance. Your body is on your side and only wishes the best for you. Sometimes we become frustrated or even angry with our bodies. I can promise in every case of your body not "cooperating," it is trying to protect you. Sometimes the body is occasionally...misguided, let's say. Help your body to heal by nurturing it with good, positive thoughts, healthy food, and joy. Surround yourself with good people. Live your life to the fullest. Have courage to step into a new world where nothing is the way it used to be. Your turn is now. Instead of fear, choose trust and curiosity—and rely on the strength within you.

In my worst moments, I felt relief in knowing I was not alone. We all face difficulties and challenges. For you, this may be a difficult divorce, your child falling ill, worries related to your parents, losing a loved one, poverty, learning difficulties...anything, really. We all get our share.

Our mind and body exist in a fully symbiotic relationship. One cannot survive without the other. It is crucial for the health of your body and mind to pay attention to the physical and mental nutrition we give ourselves during our lifetimes.

Nkosi Johnson, an AIDS activist from South Africa, put it wisely: "Do all you can with what you have, in the time you have, in the place you are." But what is it that we should do, then? The answer is simple: *pause*. At regular intervals, we should simply *pause*. That is the only way we can truly *listen*.

For me, yoga provides the best way to do this. More precisely, I have found a way to pause through yin yoga, a very slow form of yoga that involves holding *asanas* (poses) for extended periods of time, listening to the sensations in the body. There is nowhere to escape to in the yoga classes. You have no choice but to spend time in a quiet space, listening to your own body. It is common to experience new sensations, such as "Wow, I never realized that my neck was so tight," or you may have an unstoppable urge to cry and release emotion you have suppressed or have been too busy to feel and process. When we stretch our bodies at a deeper level, we begin slowly and peacefully releasing stagnations in the body. We do this with kindness and in the absence of force. We allow our bodies to let go of whatever our mind is ready to release in this very moment. Not too much and not too little.

Deep breathing exercises provide us with one extremely simple and easy way of pausing and relaxing our body. It is an unfortunate fact that in our daily lives we tend to breathe in a very superficial way, using only the upper parts of our lungs. Breathing becomes part of our daily practice. Deep breathing is calm. Calmly breathing in. Calmly breathing out. Breathing all the way down to the stomach. We can engage in deep breathing exercises wherever we go. At home, when waiting at traffic lights, or sitting at our workplaces.

Meditation has major health effects, which have also been proven by research. Meditation activates the parasympathetic nervous system in multiple ways, which is the system for calming, soothing, rest and relaxation. Among its other effects, meditation eases our mood, reduces stress, strengthens the immune system, and balances the body and mind. Meditating is also often beneficial for psychological conditions, such as insomnia, fears, and stress. A simple and easy meditation I often practice goes as follows:

I select some lovely essential oil to strengthen the impact of the meditation. I sit cross-legged (or in some other comfortable position) on a yoga mat in a place where I feel content. I straighten up my spine (perceiving my spine as my "own internal strength"), but relax all other parts of my body. This allows me to sit with good posture while being relaxed. I picture a bubble around me—my own safe space that belongs to me and me alone. I give myself this moment to take care of my wellbeing and balance. This is a moment that allows me to focus only on myself without thinking about or "helping" other people. I am within this safe bubble, perfect as I am, with all my strengths and weaknesses.

I close my eyes and calm myself by taking deeper breaths. I focus my mind on the flow of my breathing, thinking about moving in and out along with the breath. I acknowledge the distractions that may occur around me, but gently let them be. I think about leaving any external things (including thoughts, sounds, things on my to-do list) outside this bubble, this space that I inhabit. All things and thoughts can wait for me outside it. I let my breathing pass through me the way it does on this particular day, in this moment, without judgment. Without thinking "and that's good" or "that's lousy." I feel the cool air flowing in, and warm air flowing out. I feel my chest rising and falling.

I only focus my thoughts and mind on my breathing and the sensations this may cause. If my mind is restless and keeps wandering, I may count as I am breathing in (one, two, three) and out (four, five, six) and then back again. It is normal for your mind to wander, going in and out of focus. It's the nature of the mind to talk. When I catch myself doing this, I put my mind back to my breathing. However, I do this with kindness and love and without blame or shame. I am present for each of my breaths. I am present for myself. It is normal that our mind wanders to different emotions, memories, images, or plans. I let them be, and picture them leaving my body with each breath out. I let the thought or memory flow through me without getting distracted by it. I allow myself to take in the peace and good feeling the meditation gives me.

Even if one has never struggled with addiction, the Serenity Prayer from the 12-Step program Alcoholics Anonymous is helpful with illnesses of all kinds. The Serenity Prayer says: *God, grant me the serenity to accept the things I cannot change, courage to change the things I can, and the wisdom to know the difference.* I try to keep this in mind when thinking about the struggles and challenges brought by my illness. Changing what I can (doing everything in my power to heal), accepting the things I cannot change (the fact that I am living with this illness). And knowing the difference between the two (mulling over or hating the fact that I have this illness will not free me of it). I refuse to see myself as a victim; instead, I will do everything I can. I will do my best. And that is good enough.

In our hectic lives, we are not used to staying still. It comes quite naturally for us to push to our limits, sweating over things, exceeding our strengths. We will also not let ourselves slack when exercising, far from it. We may also use exercise as an escape from something (our thoughts, feeling bad, a sense of emptiness). When you are busy from morning until night, you get to ignore your thoughts and, actually, everything else.

Your whole day can be filled with busy things, starting in the morning: "Hurry, hurry, hurry! Come on, now! We're already running late! Why does it take such a long time for you to put your clothes on? Hurry up and get dressed!" We yell at our children and then step on the gas to drive to the kindergarten or school, and keep up this pace once we get to work. A cup of coffee to replace lunch, a meal poor in nutrients for lunch or skipping lunch altogether, making a stop at a grocery store on our way home from work, and then some evening chores, put the children to bed, after which we are completely and utterly beat.

Sound familiar?

It should not be this way.

We can *actually* affect our own well-being. No one else is going to do that for us. We are all personally responsible for our pace. Your boss at work won't be the one telling you to "take it easy, take as much time for this project as you like." However, to my delight, I have noticed some progress in this area. Many companies are already thinking about well-being for their entire workforce. They understand that if their employees are feeling well, their whole community thrives, which results in better quality of work and a significant reduction in sickness absences.

I know what you are thinking: it is easier said than done. What do you mean I have a say in this? The same job, same boss, same busy lifestyle—how is that going to change? I still maintain that, whether you like it or not, you *can* have a say in things if you actually want to and are willing to work on things.

Our bodies crave peace. They want us to listen to the messages they send. We should nurture our bodies: with kindness, with love. Sometimes our bodies feel tired and we should give them rest. Sometimes we are feeling fatigued, and our bodies need movement and some fresh air. We have to practice interpreting the messages correctly.

An illness is bound to change us. It hits us over the head for as long and as hard as necessary until we realize we need to pause. I am certain that my body gave me many unnoticed signs, but I had no time to stop as I was too "busy." The diagnosis I got after my first surgery was oligoastrocytoma, grade III. That was not enough. I still had too many things going on. I was in a hurry to get back to work, back to what was "normal"— in a hurry to do this, that, or the other. I did not believe it. I did not listen. And then I got another hit over the head. Grade IV. Thank you. Now I understand. I'm here and listening!

The Power of the Mind

I believe that we are not struck by an illness out of sheer coincidence. No, an illness has the purpose of letting us know that our thoughts and actions are not in balance with what is going on inside us. It is a warning, an alert. Are we living according to our values or acting against our best interests? Are we living our lives through someone else, fulfilling someone else's dreams or someone else's values? Do we keep putting ourselves last, helping other people first and ourselves after everyone else, or maybe not even then? Are we busy making sure our family is okay while giving no value to ourselves and our personal welfare?

I am a perfect example of this. I have always made sure that everyone else is doing great and seen my personal well-being as of secondary importance. I have always put my needs aside and others' needs first. We literally cannot be there for others if we are not taking care of ourselves!!

I remember my shock when I saw a talk show interviewing an aid worker helping orphan children in Russia. The person was talking about children whose mouths had been taped over at night to stop them from crying, I found it easy to feel the children's agony. I simply could not get it out of my mind. The next day, I called the telephone number of the volunteer organization. The phone call took ages. I talked and talked and talked. I talked them into taking me along to their next humanitarian aid operation. I gave no thought to when it would take place and what it would entail. All I could think about were those children. I had to get over to help them. I would not give up until the woman on the other end of the line let out a deep sigh and promised to take me along the next operation. Oh, the relief I felt. I would get to do "at least something" about it.

Time to turn my words into actions. I found myself collecting goods, cloth diapers and clothing for the children. Together with the aid workers, I packed the items into plastic bags and sacks. It was illegal to take relief goods across the Russian border. It would be considered smuggling. They'd stop us and wouldn't let us enter the country. Instead, we found a tourist bus full of young women who were going on vacation in Russia, and got a "ride" from them to St. Petersburg. At the border control we crossed our fingers, hoping they would not inspect our baggage. Apparently, we looked enough like tourists and were able to continue our trip. In St. Petersburg, we divided the bags and planned where we would each take the items. We were also helped by the organization's local volunteers. They served as our interpreters. After all, none of us knew any Russian.

I remember one giant orphanage around an hour and a half's drive from St Petersburg. They must have had 40 children. The house was in a dreadful state and covered in mold. The stench got to you right at the front door. The children were so little: from babies to around 8-year-olds. I cannot describe the sympathy and empathy I felt when I saw them. I wanted to take all of them to Finland, to be safe. The children spent most of their days sitting or lying in cribs. Now we got to pick them up from their beds to play on a carpet. We gave them toys and also took them to play outside on a run-down swing. We gave their caregivers clothing and other items. We tried our best to explain to them what a cloth diaper was and how it was used. The children's diapers were full and were only changed once per day. We were unsure about whether there was any-one to look after the children at night.

In some orphanages, the children were left alone during the night. I was most appalled by what was going on with disabled children. We only found them later, as they were segregated from these other, "normal" children. The disabled children had been completely isolated to their rooms, and left there alone. They were sitting in high chairs without mat-tresses or any sort of stimuli. They had been totally rejected and had no human contact.

When we asked the orphanage workers what was in the basement, they told us that was where they kept the babies with AIDS and we were not per-

mitted to go there. We could only imagine the condi-
tions that the babies must have endured.

I soaked in all of this pain. I could not stop think-
ing about all the evil in the world. Why will nobody
help these children? Why can we not adopt them?
Why, why, why?

When I returned back home, I wrote every mem-
ber of parliament and decision-maker I could think
of, explaining to them what I had seen during the
operation, including pictures of the children in the
letters. None of them replied to me.

You should not bottle up your emotions, you should let them out. In Finland it's very common to bottle up emotions for fear of burdening others with your worries. For the sake of healing, it's extremely important to release feelings! The only way we can reshape our thoughts and affect our emotional lives is by living through and accepting our emotions. All of our emotions and thoughts have the ability to adversely affect us at the cellular level. They shape our brains and affect many things, including the functions of our internal organs.

I believe my illness came to teach me healthy selfishness. That means I must take care of myself first and can only be of help to others through my own well-being. I also believe the people who are struck by cancer are often the ones helping others. We are those people who put themselves last in line and wish for everyone else to be okay. We are bad at asking for help. Whenever I meet someone with cancer, I say: "Hey, now is truly the time for you to think about yourself. You can accept all the help, support and love given to you. Now is your turn."

While I find it hard to be selfish, my personal values, well-being, and balance have gained a new meaning. These days, I am enjoying my life to the fullest. I go to lovely cafés and restaurants, meet my friends and laugh to my heart's content. I did all of this before, but now I feel these things more deeply. I appreciate and have gratitude. All the way at the cellular level, I feel I deserve all the good coming my way. I am able to enjoy the tiniest things.

Our minds are fully connected to our bodies. If your mind is unwell, so is your body, and vice versa. We cannot simply take a pill to counteract our symptoms; instead, we must dig deep to find the ultimate cause and root of the symptom.

A lot of the time, stress is the root cause. This may be mental or physical. Typically, an illness is the consequence of long-term mental stress or trauma. Your mind and body are simply no longer able to cope with the imbalance they are constantly being exposed to, and break into illness as if saying to you: "See me." We can imagine this is the point when our healing begins. Healing is a long, spiritual process. It is important to release yourself from your old emotional blocks, to let go of your old, rigid beliefs, and to forgive. Those of us who are too "nice" to others tend to have built-up anger, unforgiveness, and sorrow within us. We soak up the whole world's pain. We are incapable or too afraid of letting go. It is extremely important for us to cleanse our minds, let go of our emotional blocks and forgive ourselves and others. Complementary treatments, therapy, meditation and yoga may be helpful. An expert in traditional Chinese medicine put it well: "Instead of treating cancer, we are removing blockages in your health." It is essential to understand this. The road to healing and integrity is long and worthwhile.

An illness is always a sign of a lack of balance in your body. It means your body and mind are disconnected. There is a block there somewhere, preventing energy from flowing freely—and this is the source of the initial symptoms of the disease. At this point, it is worth waking up and starting to figure out where we have failed to be friends to our bodies, minds, and pain. When have we ignored the messages our bodies have been sending us?

I am sure my body had been whispering to me countless times, trying to make me understand that it was time to take a breather. Slow down! My body had to scream in order for me to listen. And it sure did, so loud I fell down!

In the fall of 2011, right before my diagnosis, I was at another hosting gig in Helsinki. All of a sudden, my right leg collapsed under me. My mind and the rest of my body worked as normal, but my leg kind of "fainted." I fell to the floor while still holding my microphone. I hallucinated that there was a person next to me. I looked over at them but saw no one. I lifted my arm towards the person, but all I could feel was the air. What was going on here?

I got up and told the salesperson standing in front of me that I slipped and fell. I continued my gig as if nothing had happened. My mind tried to make sense of it all, and I explained to myself I must have slipped somehow. After all, it was a long day and I was wearing heels. At the same time I knew I had not slipped, but had no idea what else could have been going on. I put it out of my mind.

*The next episode took place around three weeks later. I was on another hosting trip in Jyväskylä, eating at a hotel restaurant. I had ordered red wine, and just as I was trying to reach for the glass, my hand went **past** the glass. What is this, a prank? Again, I was left unable to make sense of what had happened.*

The worst episode occurred in Tampere, just as I was driving 130 km/h on the highway. All of a sudden, I had a total blackout. I had no idea how to drive. I no longer knew which pedal was the brake, which was the gas. I just drew a complete blank. In my state of shock, I pressed all the buttons I could see at the same time. The car made a terrible sound. God, please help me—let me get back home alive!

By some miracle, I was able to get back home. This was the first time I told my husband, Jussi, about the strange symptoms I had been having. I was shaking. Together, we decided we had to get to the bottom of it.

I booked an appointment with a neurologist. I told the doctor about my symptoms, and they just told me that what I was probably experiencing was a migraine. The spectrum of migraine is so wide that the symptoms may be exactly like the ones I had experienced. I was given anti-migraine drugs, which I was never planning to take. At this point, my intuition was telling me (screaming at me, really) that what I was experiencing was definitely not a migraine. Even though I had no idea what exactly I was having, I knew for sure that this was not it.

Of course, I kept having the symptoms, and three months after the first appointment, I booked a new one with a different neurologist. That was Valentine's Day 2012, the day I got my correct diagnosis.

Stress is the worst enemy of the immune system. Our bodies whisper to us when we are heading in the wrong direction and not living our lives according to our core values and engaging in things that are not healthy for us. These whispers may take the form of headaches, back pain, rhinitis, sinusitis, eye infections, hives, fatigue, exhaustion, insomnia, stress, or an urge to fill our time with constant activity. The question is: are we listening? If we are always busy and cram our lives full of stressful activities, occupy ourselves in the rat race at a constantly accelerating rate, spend our days compulsively engaging in things we feel like we just have to do, the answer is no—we are not listening. We are ignoring all the little cues our bodies give us to make us listen, kindly and with love. We neglect a headache by promptly taking a painkiller; we avoid insomnia by taking melatonin or a sleeping pill—we numb the symptom. Which, quite obviously, does nothing to the actual cause. It only makes it worse. Stress increases our blood glucose concentration, and chronic stress increases it, well, chronically. If cancer cells feed off of sugar, this helps us understand how stress contributes to cancer.

The amygdala, located in our brain, acts as a kind of an alarm system warning us when we are facing impending danger. It identifies the threat and sends a warning to the thalamus. The thalamus, located in the center of the brain, sends a signal to the brain stem. The sympathetic nervous system sends signals to all the major organs and muscle groups in the body, preparing them for a fight-flight-or-freeze situation. The hypothalamus signals the pituitary gland to alert the adrenal glands to produce stress hormones: adrenaline and cortisol. Cortisol and stress also raise blood glucose levels, as glucose is necessary for the fight-flight-or-freeze response. This makes our hearts beat faster (to bring more blood in the body and improve our functional ability), pupils dilate (to allow your eyes collect more light), and lungs work more efficiently, improving the oxygen supply to the brain. This allows us to fight or run away as fast as we can, or simply freeze and not move so we remain undetected by a predator.

When you are having an epileptic seizure, the fight-flight-or-freeze response starts immediately. The heart starts beating extremely fast, palms are sweaty and the whole body is in a severe state of stress. Even though you cannot think clearly, your body starts working on autopilot, preparing for protective measures.

It is incomprehensible what this feels like in practice. When an epileptic seizure strikes, I do not freeze from terror—I act. I am terrified, but I take action. After each episode, I am absolutely beat. All I want to do is sleep. And when I wake up, I am ravenously hungry. This shows you how taxing and stressful the fight-flight-or-freeze response always is. I am sure everyone can think of similar situations in their lives.

One time, I was on my way to host an event in Lahti. I jumped on a train in Tampere and was supposed to change to another train traveling towards Lahti in Riihimäki. Right at the start of my journey, I started having the strangest feeling: confusion, fear and loss of consciousness. I felt as if my heart was beating in my arm. I knew I was about to have an epileptic seizure. I froze on the spot. I knew I had little time to act. Who could I talk to about this? What would I say? I was going to have to change trains in Riihimäki. I got up and started looking for a conductor, and was able to find one quickly. I explained to them as clearly as I could what was about to happen. I also told them I was going to have to change trains in Riihimäki and get to the train heading for Lahti. I felt the throbbing on my arm rising up, towards my right ear. I ran back to my seat. I emptied an oral syringe of Epistatus solution into my mouth. I fell asleep very quickly.

I only have faint recollections of the rest of my journey. In some way or other, the conductor had been able to make me get up in Riihimäki, where I staggered along the train hallway and to the other train. I was completely out of it because of the medication.

I should obviously not have gone anywhere on my own at that point. I would have needed someone to escort me to the train. I forgot to mention this to the conductor. The next thing I remember is walking unsteadily on a street in Lahti. There was a jolly group of women next to me who had clearly been spending their day in a bar. They made lots of noise, talking loudly and laughing rowdily. I remember asking them which way I should go to find my hotel. The words that came out of my mouth were like a drunk person's slurred speech. The women laughed at my confused state but told me where to go. I have a vague recollection of signing in to a hotel at the front desk. I remember realizing that my handwriting was so messy it made no sense to anyone. But I chose not to explain any of this to the receptionist as I was also struggling to speak.

Being the diligent worker that I am, I set my alarm clock for eight am the next morning—and went to my hosting gig as if nothing had happened.

If our body is in a chronic state of emergency, our own defense system begins gradually losing its grip, eventually weakening our immune system. Little by little, the amygdala starts to react more sensitively to even minor threats, such as thoughts, beliefs, memories, and traumas. Constant, chronic stress throws us off balance and starts affecting our health.

The opposite of these mechanisms is found in the parasympathetic nervous system, which has the purpose of bringing balance and stability to the body and mind. The parasympathetic nervous system's job is to create a sense that everything is fine. We need both of these systems: the sympathetic and parasympathetic nervous system. They go hand in hand to keep us alive.

Cellular memory is an interesting scientific concept. The cells store information, memories and traumas from our childhood, as well as the lives of our parents and grandparents. Memories have been found to transcend generations. This particularly applies to traumatic memories of fears. The emerging scientific field of Epigenetics is currently investigating how trauma leaves a chemical "mark" on DNA, and can be passed to our biological offspring. This means it truly matters how we treat our own and our inherited traumas and memories. Even just acknowledging all of this helps us better understand our parents and our entire family history. It is extremely important we stop the transfer of negative experiences to the next generation, our own children. We can do this through awareness and by taking good care of ourselves.

I cannot help but think how positive emotions and experiences of success already affect us in early childhood, influencing children's immune system, as well as their self-esteem and mind. These days, whenever I meet my children's teachers at parent-teacher conferences, I always point out that, as a mother, I believe it is most important to give our children positive feedback and ensure they have experiences of success. Having masterful experiences has been proven to increase children's feelings of self-efficacy, and also they learn that "failure" is simply a part of the mastery process. "Failure" at a task does not mean the child themselves is a failure, nor does it mean that success is impossible in the future. This is more important than exam results or scholarships. If a child is doing their best, it is enough. It must be enough. I hope schools can receive more resources to allow them to take every child's special needs into account and see all children as individuals and perfect just the way they are—with all their strengths and weaknesses.

In other words, everything we do matters. Healing is a far more complex process than we have dared to imagine. It is not easy, but it is possible.

The Importance of Hope for Healing

Dominique Surel is a researcher at Harvard investigating the psychological effects of placebo on healing. In her studies, she has explored something I have always known based on my intuition: the *way* doctors tell their patients about a cancer diagnosis, whether giving them hope and encouragement or giving this as a sort of death sentence without any hope, has a significant impact on the patient's healing or not healing.

Giving a patient a poor prognosis in a matter-of-fact way may make the patient feel completely terrified and hopeless. As a result, the person may start living their lives "according to their cancer grade." If a doctor gives the patient a prognosis "from a few months to a year at best," the patient will be left with no hope. In fact, the prognosis will all but destroy any shred of hope the patient may have had up until this point. **Patients have the right to receive truthful information about their illness and its severity. But they must not lose all hope.** This is why I am convinced doctors should not give a life expectancy to patients unless the patient expressly states an interest in knowing. The fact is, no doctor can know for sure how things will actually go. Nobody knows!

I remember one male physician who ironically smirked at me when I asked him about my possibilities for healing from my cancer: "Well, I mean, if you're still sitting across from me in five years, I'll give you a clean bill of health."

A doctor can do an incredible job at helping and supporting a patient simply by saying, "We will do everything in our power for you to get better." This is not a promise that you will heal—but it gives you hope.

Once, I asked a doctor about this and she told me, "We shouldn't give you any false hope." *What* exactly is false hope? Am I supposed to simply act out my fate and start planning my own funeral? I understand doctors are unable to give you an unfounded promise that you will get better if your prospects are extremely poor. But even in such cases, they could give you information about complementary therapies outside the field of medicine, such as oxygen therapy, juicing, or clinics offering holistic cancer care. Give nature a chance to do its thing. What is there to lose? I personally believe each one of us would rather live their final years, months, or weeks in hope rather than despair.

After my second surgery, I had an MRI scheduled every three months. This was an endless source of anxiety for me: *what if it's there again...* Constant fear of the tumor recurring. I'd experience such an amazing sense of relief when the doctor said the images came back normal. After each time, I was able to go back to living my life, feeling relieved for the following 1.5 months, after which my anxiety for the next MRI started building up. My life followed these cycles. Anxiety, relief, anxiety, relief.

One time, I remember seeing an oncologist for the results

of another MRI. This time, I met with a cancer specialist I had never seen before. The doctor looked at me with a puzzled expression (I could tell they expected me to look different—like someone who had my diagnosis, ie. a half-dead person). The doctor looked at their computer screen, then back to me, and again looked at the computer screen. I could see they were dying to ask me "are you sure you are the person this text refers to?" There I sat in front of them, doing well and carrying a yoga mat with me. The magnetic images were healthy. No growth or changes. Just as I was leaving the appointment, the doctor told me something I will never forget: **"I don't know what you're doing, but keep doing whatever it is!"**

Even if we are genetically predisposed to some diseases does not mean that those genes will actually be triggered and we are bound to fall ill. One can have the genes for illness, mental or physical, and simply lack the environmental conditions necessary to activate those genes. Hence, they never get sick. We should instead think that having this potentially bigger illness risk gives us a reason to pay more attention to our lifestyles and diets, and make sure we are not living in constant stress. What we have to change is our *thinking* about getting an illness. It is important not to be overcome by fear. After all, stress contributes more to diseases than the genes we happen to have.

The inherited BRCA gene is a good example of this. Many women have had a mastectomy after learning they carry a mutated BRCA gene, which is linked to increased breast cancer risk. The reason for this is simple: fear. People start living according to their fear. They start thinking they are going to get breast cancer when they carry this particular gene. We let fear control us, even though what we should be doing is to pay slightly more attention to what our lifestyles are like, how we eat and engage in physical activity. Are our lives in balance? I do not think it is beneficial to start fearing something we do not even have yet—and may never even have.

Previous studies have compared the lifestyles of nearly five hundred sets of twins. It has been observed lifestyles have far greater health impacts than genes. Out of a set of twins with identical genes, one might fall ill and the other live a fully healthy life. It all depends on lifestyle choices: what you consume and how you live. Even if a lot of people in your family have cancer and your genes are considered high risk, you can affect your health through your own actions. Perhaps you need to be more deliberate about it, but it is still fully possible. The power lies in our hands, on our plates, and in our minds.

The good thing is that our cells are constantly renewing. This means our bodies are rebuilding themselves all the time. Our bodies are naturally predisposed to finding balance, homeostasis. At a point when we fall ill, our bodies are already in a state of emergency. At all times, our bodies aim to find a path towards healing. Our bodies want to heal. Let's give them the chance to do just that.

I fully believe our minds can make us ill, but they can also heal us. What is the story you tell yourself? Do you see yourself as a victim, to whom only bad things happen? Are you someone who always gets the short end of the stick? Or do you believe everything happens for a reason, and the crises in our lives are, in fact, the times when we grow the most? Chögyam Trungpa Rinpoche, a Tibetan Buddhist leader, described the experience of crisis opening us up as "shaky tenderness." These are turning points allowing us to look at the track we are on and decide which way to turn.

Our emotions and thoughts have a major impact on our illness—and on our healing. What are your beliefs about yourself? Do you perceive yourself as a beautiful, thriving, and healthy person, or do you feel sorry for yourself and always find something negative and bad to say about yourself? It's been proven that stress is only harmful when we perceive it negatively, or beyond our ability to manage. Otherwise, stress has many benefits, including immunity boosting and making us more resilient.

You can always choose. You can choose health. '

After my second operation, I decided that I was going to start living now. To do all the things I always wanted. Right now! Not later.

After I had said goodbye to a year of cytostatic therapy and decided to give my body the peace and space it needed for healing itself, I made the choice to go on a yoga retreat, on my own. This was a major step on my road to recovery. For a long time, I had been following the writings of yoga instructor Satu Tuomela on social media. Even though I had never actually met her, I decided to participate in her *This is Where the Magic Happens* retreat. The retreat took place in Santorini, Greece. This week turned out to be a major turning point for me.

Before this, I never realized what poor shape my body was in. My legs were shaking so much I had trouble standing up. I kept wondering what all these other people, undoubtedly top yogis, would think about me, a person unable to perform the easiest balancing poses without wobbling. But I tried my best. I tried even though I was trembling. I rested if I had to, and continued as soon as I could find the strength. I decided the only way for me was forward. I got to know the most wonderful people at the retreat. With them, I spent time at the pool, had dinners in the evenings, and laughed to my heart's content.

I fell head over heels in love with yin yoga. It felt like my thing right away. It was so therapeutic and peaceful, something my soul and heart had been craving for a long time. I had not known such a wonderful thing existed.

On the day before leaving the retreat, I realized I had not called home *even once*. It was completely unheard of and totally unlike me. But this was a sign. Now, perhaps for the first time in my life, I was able to leave everything behind and surrender myself fully to the present moment.

I struggled a lot with going back to my old daily life after the retreat. It was like stepping onto a different planet. I felt the exact same thing as when I had left the hospital: nothing in the outside world had changed, but nothing was the same for me.

About six months after the retreat, I got an email from Satu, who was the instructor. In her message, she wrote that she was starting a yoga instructor course with a small group. Less than ten students would be enrolled in the course. She thought I would be one of them. I kept rereading the message, certain she had accidentally sent this email to the wrong person. I could not imagine she was actually asking me to take part in the training.

Me, who could not even stand on one leg without trembling. *Me*, who had brain cancer. *Me*, with just one week's experience of yin yoga. I was flabbergasted. It was unbelievable.

I thought it over for about a week. I mostly pondered whether I could do it or not, if I was too weak. After all, the training was going to include 200 hours of asana practices, meditation, assisting, anatomy and physiology, the human energy system, *Prāṇāyāma* (breathing exercises), meditation, mantras and philosophy.

I messaged Satu: yes, count me in. That ended up being one of the best decisions I have ever made in my life.

Illness is a long process enabling profound spiritual growth. There is no going back to how things used to be. **Cancer is**

an invitation to change by way of your body, mind, and soul. Instead of fighting and resisting, you must harness all your inner strength to begin and maintain rebuilding. You must start the greatest love affair you have ever had in your life: the one you have with yourself.

The yoga philosophy includes an idea that each breath is an opportunity for starting your life over. We do not have to stick to our old, rigid beliefs or society's expectations. We must want to and dare to make a change.

The world is full of people who have recovered from illnesses thought to be incurable. Why are these people not written about in newspapers? Why is medicine not interested in studying these cases? And, above all: what have these people done differently than others? My life expectancy was from a few months to a year. If I had known this from the start, I am not sure I would still be here. Would my mind have "killed me" by completely discouraging me?

I started searching for people around the world who had either healed or were still living after being diagnosed with a severe form of cancer, particularly malignant brain tumor. I found glioblastoma patients who had lived for two or three years. Not good enough. I was desperate to find someone who had survived several years longer than I had.

Finally, I found someone. The last week of writing this book, a message popped into my email. It was from Yaron Butterfield, a Canadian who had been diagnosed with glioblastoma in 2004 and was doing well. I jumped for joy. This was exactly what I had been looking for.

Yaron is also a cancer researcher, working in the field of genomics. I had to find out what he had done for his healing—what were the medical treatments and complementary therapies he had used. His tumor had been inoperable at every point. He had undergone the standard radiotherapy and cytostatic therapy with temozolomide. After all of this, his tumor recurred, and a decision was made to give him new, experimental treatment. This had not worked—instead, the tumor doubled in size. He then made the decision to undergo the same cytostatic therapy again. And then something miraculous happened. After eight months of cytostatic agents, one week per month, his tumor began gradually decreasing in size. He has no further treatment for the cancer since 2006.

Yaron emphasized the fact the cytostatic drugs work differently on different individuals. Cancer originates from DNA mutations, and as every person has different DNA, we cannot know for sure what will or will not work for someone. For some individuals, certain cytostatic agents will be highly effective, while for others, the same substances might not work or even make cancer worse.

This is what also happened to me after radiotherapy. The surgeons were able to remove the visible part of the tumor in the operation. Of course, doctors and surgeons are eager to point out that it is never possible to get rid of all cancer cells, meaning some will always remain in the body. But my tumor recurred straight after radiotherapy, even though only a few months had passed after the operation. This does not mean what did not work for me could not work for somebody else.

What Yaron did for his recovery:

He kept hope up.

He believed deeply in his own recovery.

He trusted medicine and new treatments.

He used complementary therapies to support his medical treatment.

He found a peer support group which allowed him to share his experiences and get support from other people living with the same challenge.

He received support from his friends and family.

He looked to his daughter, who made him feel it was his responsibility to do everything in his power to heal from his illness. He wanted to be healthy and enjoy every moment he could with her.

He ate healthy food and kept physically active.

He did positive things and helped others.

He tried new things to help with neuroplasticity.

He gave himself a reason he needed to *live.*

If we do not know for sure how things are going to go, let us assume that everything will end up well.
– Mauno Koivisto, the ninth President of Finland

The Power of Nature

Opposing forces sustain our lives: day and night, light and darkness, warmth and coldness, strength and weakness, joy and sorrow, and, indeed, also sickness and health.

The more we develop our awareness and knowledge of our bodies, the stronger our immunity. Our bodies love the attention we give them. Diseases usually originate from a time when we have not been present in or for our bodies. We give ourselves no time to feel anything; our emotions are trampled by mindless activity. We need to listen to the whispers of our body—tension in the neck, for example, is your body's quiet request for attention and care. It will get worse if you don't tend to it.

Examples:

- If you sit at a chair all day at work, take a 2-minute stretching break every hour.
- If you stand all day, get shoes that support you better.
- If you don't sleep well or wake up at 3am to worry about work—it's your body telling you that you need a break!

Yoga helps with feeling and seeing everything more clearly. Starting yoga with breathing exercises allows us to feel the flow of our breathing, to feel the earth on which we sit and the air we breathe, hear the sounds close to and far from us, identify the scents around us, and sense all of the energy of the people we share space with.

When engaging in a sun salutation, for instance, as I am lifting up my arms, I visualize picking up energy from the ground, then from the air and sky, and finally, bringing it all to myself. I am part of all this.

As I lie on my back, I can sense every part of my body, paying attention to my toes, the bottoms of my feet, the front of my legs. I continue my observations up my legs, from my knees to my thighs and so on. I feel the energy flowing through my body.

Our bodies seek balance. Not too much or too little of anything.

Sometimes you need distance to see what is right in front of you. My disease has taught me to take care of myself. To give myself time to do things that resonate with and are important to me. And I have learned to do that without feeling guilty.

In Western countries, it is common to treat only the symptoms of disease. When we feel pain, we take a pill, and the pain will go away. We focus on the symptom instead of the cause. As a result, I have been very interested in the traditional medicine of the East on my personal healing path: Ayurveda (which originates from India), traditional Tibetan medicine, and Chinese medicine. While I am by no means a professional when it comes to these, the idea of treating people as a whole feels right to me. Instead of treating the symptoms, these forms of medicine involve going deeper, to the root cause of the problem. This requires a lot more than popping a pain pill.

Because of my outlook, I meet with the best doctors and healers whenever I am on a yoga retreat. I have been to a yoga retreat in India four years in a row now. The first one was by yoga instructor Tara Judelle and took place in Goa. The retreat was organized at the Samata Holistic Retreat Center, where food was prepared from ingredients picked from the center's organic garden. The center carries out very important work, encouraging and training villagers to use herbs and grow their own food. I was very impressed by their passion for helping and their focus on making the world a better place, one village at a time. Their clinic was also where I met Eric Rosenbush, a medical practitioner specializing in Ayurvedic and Tibetan medicine. He offers Ayurvedic consultations, healing and acupuncture. He provided me with a lot of information and herbs collected from the Himalayas with health-balancing properties. These herbs and the different treatments I received have been extremely important to me.

After this initial visit, I could not help but keep returning to India. I studied chakras and healing under Didier Fernandes and Alicia Pulgarcita. In the Summer of 2017, I was invited to the Yoga Ambassador tour in Kerala, India. This was a no-cost and truly amazing adventure across the beautiful state of Kerala. I felt so privileged to have been chosen for this unbelievable journey. India has taught me about the power inherent in nature.

Nature has everything we need for healing. The knowledge that the local people have of the healing powers of spices and plants, for instance, is mind-blowing. Some time after this trip, I returned to India for yoga instructor training. This time, my main instructors were Yamuna Devi and Tobie Tomkinton. In addition, Matthew Clark taught us philosophy. I could have spent ages listening to his stories. Among his many experiences, he had lived with isolated tribes in India and Africa and explored life in tribal cultures. He also taught me about the connection we have with nature: with rocks, trees, earth, plants, water, and animals. We are all truly one.

The Sanskrit word *ayur-veda* means knowledge of life: the connection between the body and the mind, as well as the physical teachings of Ayurveda, such as diets and lifestyles based on each bodily humor. According to Ayurveda, humans can achieve perfect health and life by following three elements: the correct diet, the correct lifestyle, and the correct thoughts—based on each individual's bodily humor.

Ayurveda aims to guide people to live in balance with themselves and nature. It has a multi-faceted approach: internal and external, emotional and spiritual. We eat healthy and high-quality food. We maintain healthy and balanced interpersonal relationships. We live out our own unique personal potential and meaning to the maximum, in harmony with the purpose of the entire universe.

If we want to understand the principles of Ayurveda, we simply need to look at the seasonal changes in nature. We see the impacts of three forces—water energy, fire energy and air energy. It would take a full book to fully explain all of this; in fact, plenty of books are available on the topic. Nevertheless, I want to point out some very basic aspects of Ayurveda in this section, as I have strong faith in this ancient and wise form of medicine and its potential for helping us take care of our health and treat our illnesses.

It is a good idea to start by determining your dominant type and spend some time reading up on it. There are three elemental bodily humors, or doshas: Vata, Pitta and Kapha. I am a combination of two doshas, Vata and Pitta, of which Vata is more dominant.

A special guide to Ayurveda is below!

Vata reflects the element of air. Nothing in nature can survive without air. Each breath sustains our life, or prana. Vata creates movement in nature, all living creatures, and inanimate objects on earth. At a symbolic level, Vata signifies change. It teaches us nothing is permanent.

Vata is strongest in the early hours of the morning from

2–6AM and in the afternoons from 2–6PM. Vata's movements affect the systems of our bodies and minds. Inward moving strength allows our bodies to perform vital functions, such as swallowing food, obtaining and distributing nutrition to different tissues, and receiving oxygen. At the level of the mind, this inward movement of air allows the brain to comprehend the received information, transforming thoughts to feelings, and feelings to emotions.

In turn, the outward energy of Vata allows the body to flush out metabolic waste and toxins as well as sweat, urine, and mucus. Vata means fast metabolism. It helps the body release old cells. It supports bodily functions, particularly basic motor functions, including coordinated movements of legs, arms and head, and all muscles of the face, fingers and toes, and stretching of muscles. At the level of the mind, this outward energy allows us to quickly recall the details of some memory which, in turn, enables us to react to what other people say or do. At the physical level, Vata is located in the lower abdomen in the human body. In this area, the element regulates the genitals as well as the large intestine and the rectum.

Vata imbalance often manifests in the pelvis region, on the knees, and as stiffness of muscles and joints. It often results in coldness and dryness of the skin. You may experience digestive issues, diseases of the prostate or ovaries, menstrual problems, or miscarriages. At the level of the mind, a Vata imbalance results in mind-wandering, feelings of fear, nightmares, difficulties falling asleep, and worrying. As Vata is a cold element, it is easy to determine its state in the body and mind. An imbalance may be apparent as a blueness of skin and nails, dryness of skin and hair, and skin ulcers.

When our Vata is in balance, we are physically active and get enough rest. We are creative, restful and balanced at the same time. If our dominant biological energy (or element) is Vata, we should avoid eating bitter-tasting foods (especially during cold seasons). Here in Finland, a Vata-dominant person is always bound to feel cold, and needs to keep their woolly knit socks on at all times.

Dryness and poor nutrition are the biggest health issues for those with a dominant Vata dosha. If your dominant dosha is Vata, you should eat food that is full of nutrients and keeps you full. Those with Vata dominance tend to have a craving for warm meals (as your body is cold). The more I have learned to listen to my body, the more I have realized that my body will tell me what is good for it. For example, I have never been able to get into a raw food diet or eating salads. I feel food like that never satisfies me enough and always leaves my body feeling cold. This is also a reason why warm vegetarian dishes are ideal for me.

When Vata is your dominant element, fats with high warmth and moisture content are good for you: butter and ghee, and olive, almond, sesame, avocado and flaxseed oil. You should opt for sweet-tasting fruit: banana, fresh dates and figs, mango, grapes, lime, lemon, papaya, apricots, straw-berries, raspberries and blueberries. While nuts and seeds are good for the Vata, you should eat them in moderation to prop-erly digest them. Because those of us with Vata dominance have to deal with dryness, we also need to drink more than the Pitta and Kapha types.

Pitta is a fire energy, so naturally it dominates during sun hours, midday and midnight. At the symbolic level, Pitta sig-nifies power and strength. A Pitta person is characterized by a tidy and well-organized nature. Pitta controls seasonal varia-tion and earth with the power of heat and light. Pitta includes heat-producing characteristics, which are necessary for pro-viding energy for reproduction and regeneration.

In the human body, Pitta leads the blood circulation to ensure the flow of nutrients to cells and maintenance of the body's central system. The fire of Pitta influences the area of the stomach and is linked to the digestive process by affecting the acids that allow the body to digest food. Pitta helps the ab-sorption of nutrients, minerals, vitamins and fatty acids. This is vital for sustaining health.

Pitta regulates our body temperature. When we have fe-ver or other diseases, our body temperature rises to provide the immune system with as much strength to heal as possi-ble. Pitta also regulates white and red blood cells, controls the immune system, and aids blood coagulation capacity. Pitta guides the pores in opening and closing to regulate our body temperature.

When Pitta is in balance, our digestion is working, our memory is sharp, we are patient, and talk and act efficiently. Pitta imbalance, by contrast, leads to digestive issues, weakens our immune system and blood values, and increases stress. We are angry, stressed, and unsatisfied. This may also be physically visible: as ulcers, skin issues (such as chapping and psoriasis), or tumors, especially ones located in the stomach, liver and pancreas.

If you are "hot-blooded," sweat a lot, your body feels warm, your cheeks are flushed or your eyes red, then your body has excess Pitta. Pitta-dominant individuals need calming and cooling foods and drinks. They have high blood acidity, and should therefore avoid eating meat.

The ideal diet for Pitta types is calming and cooling, not too high in fat. Pitta individuals are advised to reduce the "fire and heat" in their bodies, and should therefore favor sweet and mild spices, such as fennel, clove, caraway, dill, turmeric, mint, and rosemary. The best nuts and seeds for these individuals are sunflower seeds and pumpkin seeds, but should be eaten in moderation. Pitta individuals should favor a diet rich in root vegetables and other plants.

Kapha is water energy. It is most potent in the mornings at 6–10AM and early evenings at 6–10PM.

Excessive Kapha prevents prana (energy) from flowing freely. Your heart pumps blood to your different body parts. A constant flow is a sign of health, while obstructions in this will lead to diseases. The same goes for everything in life, including relationships. We also want a freely moving flow in our relationships.

At the level of the mind, your Kapha is imbalanced if you are too attached to people or material things. Kapha individuals should usually exercise some discipline in limiting the amounts of food they consume. Products of animal origin, such as eggs, meat and dairy products, are least suitable for Kapha individuals. Kapha-dominant people do not need a lot of fat and fatty foods. Instead, they are recommended to consume ginger, garlic, curry and dill, and vegetables such as spinach, arugula, broccoli, beetroot, Brussels sprouts, eggplant and salads.

If your dominant element is Kapha, you should also include beans, red and yellow lentils, and mung beans in your diet. You should also drink tea, particularly ginger tea and green tea, which remove toxins.

The body and mind are fully connected: when your mind is healthy, your body is also healthy. What we eat, how we live, and what goes on in our minds lays the foundation for the health of our bodies and minds.

Janesh Vadya, a famous Ayurveda practitioner told me that even if 99% of your life seems to be completely covered in darkness with no way out, at least 1% will always be full of light and good. You should work your way towards that 1%. Towards the light. This was a teaching given to Janesh by his grandparents. It is a great piece of advice for us all.

In another life, I worked for a few years as a flight attendant for the Finnair airline. This had been my childhood dream job—after all, I always loved traveling and seeing different countries. I also liked the irregularity of the job.

So here I was, working in my dream job, and yet I had a feeling as if someone was choking me. Why could I not be happy? After all, finding a permanent job is like winning the lottery these days. Of course, I enjoyed seeing countries I wouldn't necessarily get to see otherwise. I worked on many red-eye flights. It was not uncommon to fly to the destination overnight and then go and see whatever city I was in straight after landing (whether it be in China, Japan or India). In the evening, I collapsed into bed, tired as a zombie, only to wake up very early for the return flight. Once I got back to Finland, I hopped on the bus heading to Tampere, and then had to travel an additional 30 minutes to my home to see my little children who had been missing me tremendously. I was completely beat, but also had to muster up the energy to do things at home. I also felt guilty about having spent time away. I did not find the pace of this lifestyle suitable for me in any way, shape, or form. My body was in constant overdrive and I was always in a state of stress. After a few years at my job, I resigned. When I listened to the depths of my soul and my personal values, I realized that this dream job was not the right thing for me, after all.

Now that I have been studying all of these things related to healing and health, I have also come to understand how unhealthy it is to make your body act against its internal clock.

It is extremely important for us to take care of ourselves and others. To treat ourselves and others as we would want to be treated. Everything begins with feeling good and having a good relationship with yourself. Only when you have this sorted out can you be honestly present in your other relationships—including those with people, animals and nature.

Asylum seekers began arriving in Finland in great numbers in the fall of 2015. I immediately felt a great need to do something, anything at all, to help them. Even though I knew my input would only be a drop in the ocean, I could not just stand there and do nothing. I asked my friend Gil to join me. I had known them since school and knew we shared the same values and they would be eager to help. We went to work the night shift at an emergency unit operated by the Finnish Red Cross. I ended up working at the reception center. What pulled me there was simply my empathy and desire to help. When the first busload of families arrived, full of little children who were hungry, cold and frightened, I could sense the agony and fear of each and every one of them. I felt discouraged taking them to cold, empty rooms with nothing more than beds on the floor. It was December and so dark you could not see in front of you. But these children were just like anyone else here in Finland. They all had their dreams and wishes, even though these were distant from those of their Western peers about new phones and vacations. All these children wished for was safety. They wished that they would not have to see another loved one be killed. And yet: they were full of joy. I could not have felt more empathy towards these children. I wanted to give them something, anything, just a pinch of trust in life.

There is nothing wrong with wanting good things for your-self, similarly as you might wish for good things to happen to those close to you or someone you don't even know. There is nothing wrong with wishing for good health, strength, and balance. I wish to stay healthy for many, many years. I want to see my children grow up, find their own paths in life, some-one to share their lives with. I want to continue being happy, balanced, and empathetic. And I want that for each and every person.

I believe we have a much deeper connection with animals than we even realize. A few years ago, my family was vaca-tioning in Thailand. On the small island of Puda, we came across an absolutely delightful monkey. You could see from miles away what a gentle animal this was. Our Nooa, the brave one that he is, went to get to know the monkey right away. He threw the monkey a water bottle filled with seawater. The monkey pulled the cork out of the bottle with its teeth, smelled that it was seawater, cast Nooa an angry glance and threw the bottle away. Nooa immediately understood that the monkey obviously needed proper drinking water, went to pick a water bottle for the monkey, and handed the bottle to the monkey. The monkey seemed elated and drank the entire bottle of wa-ter, turned towards Nooa and nodded with glee, as if to thank him. Then he came and sat down right next to Nooa and start-ed grooming Nooa's hair and scratching his head, as if to show him his gratitude. After around 10 minutes of doing this, the monkey stopped what it was doing, leaned back and closed its eyes. For a moment, we were wondering what was going to happen next. And then, Nooa realized that it was now his turn to start grooming and scratching the monkey. Oh, the look of pleasure on the monkey's face when Nooa was petting it! This is a lovely story of the similarity of humans and animals.

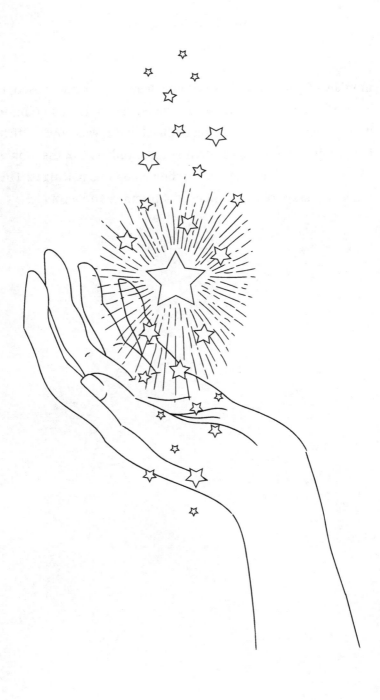

OUR PERSONAL RESPONSIBILITY FOR HEALING

I t absolutely amazes me what a spiritual world opened up as a result of this illness. I finally understand: I am not *just* my physical body (legs, hands, fingers, brain...). Alongside this, there is my energy body, which is at least as important as the physical body.

I believe that energy medicine will gain prominence as an area of medicine in the future. According to Albert Szent-Györgyi, a Nobel laureate in Medicine, "in every culture and in every medical tradition before ours, healing was accomplished by moving energy." Energy medicine is a science of physical, psychological, and spiritual health and vitality. In practice, this means an ability to perceive our bodies as a living energy system, whose balance we can influence with our everyday choices. Energy medicine refers to a harmony of the body, mind, and soul.

I started looking for stories of healing from around the world. One of the people I found was Donna Eden, who talks about her healing process in her book, Energy Medicine: Balancing Your Body's Energies for Optimal Health, Joy, and Vitality. When she was born, she was diagnosed with a heart murmur, contracted tuberculosis as a child, and had numerous food allergies. She later presented with the initial symptoms of MS, got asthma when she was in her late twenties, and a tumor was found in her breast. Simply put, all her physical systems were failing. Her doctors had already given up and told her "to put her things in order." She retreated to Fiji to live a very simple life. She and her family lived in the wilderness, far from the nearest town. Every day, she went swimming in the ocean, ate breadfruit that had fallen on the ground and fish caught from the ocean. None of her food was processed. None of it came ready-made in a jar or packaging. All of it was fresh, organic food. There were no cars emitting exhaust gases or chemical substances dusting from clothing. No competition or stress or any pressure for achieving things. And she regained her health, simply by living naturally.

I love stories like these. I also started reading a lot about Chinese medicine. How the meridians, chakras and stagnations (energy blockages) in our bodies affect our health or illness. A cancerous tumor is simply a mass of pent-up energy. It is a blockage preventing free energy flow. All of this points out how very important it is that our emotions and thoughts are in harmony with our personal values. We must think positively, and ensure the energy flowing through our bodies is strong. This allows us to stay healthy.

No single aspect will suffice on its own: not just diet, vitamins, positive thoughts, yoga, green smoothies, not just radiotherapy. Nothing is enough on its own. What we have to do instead is to create something much broader, a Healing Circle. What we need is a lot of motivation, positivity, belief in ourselves and our possibilities for healing, and also the courage to feel weak and ask others for help. It is also important to notice the thinking patterns and beliefs we may be carrying with ourselves. We need courageousness to dive deep into the origins of the disease.

Every day we make hundreds, if not thousands, of decisions. I try to make tiny little changes which support, rather than corrupt, my personal journey. Below are some of my recommendations for you:

- Trade all synthetic substances you use, such as cosmetics and cleaning agents, for natural products. Simply get rid of all synthetic toxic agents and chemicals in your home. Around 60% of the products we use are absorbed into our circulation system. At such a high rate, you will want all the products you use to be nourishing and completely non-toxic. You should only put things on your skin you would not think twice about eating. For example, coconut oil works well as a lotion for your skin. It works both internally and externally. It is also a lovely lotion for children.

- Engage in deep breathing and get fresh outdoor air. This allows your soul and mind to feel restful. It is the best kind of stress removal, calming your entire body.

- Introduce yoga or some other calming routine as part of your everyday life. You may include some lovely music that empowers you, or choose to practice in complete silence. This routine can also be something else, such as a walk in a forest. It can be anything that makes you feel that your nervous system is restful.

- Spend time with the people who are important to you. Who are Your People?

- Eat food that is as clean as possible. Trade the products you use for organic ones.

- Believe in your ability to heal. If you do not believe in it, no one else will. Do not listen to life expectancy predictions. No one can truly know how much time you have left. Trust in your intuition and strengthen its power. Build good relationships with the doctors in charge of your care and nursing staff. Value their truly important work. Let them know that you appreciate their work. They are part of your path towards healing.

- Stop and listen to what kind of a person you are *today*. It is so common for us to stay in that old, familiar rat race like we always have done instead of stepping out of it to think about how we have actually changed. What kind of a person am I right *now*? What are my values and dreams today? Who are the people that mean the most to me, who are the ones I would most like to spend my time with? What does my body need for healing?

Research has indicated that feeling helpless, or seeing yourself as a victim, has the tendency of reducing our immunity and shortening our lifespan. We may then ask that if a sense of helplessness reduces our potential for healing, what is the effect of its opposite, a sense of *control*—a feeling that *I am taking personal responsibility* for my own health?

I try to listen to myself as well as I can and live accordingly. I wake up without hurry, in tune with my internal and circadian rhythm. I breathe in fresh air. I am grateful that this is possible for me. Not many people can regulate their schedules and enjoy peaceful mornings.

Think about what rhythm in your life would suit you the best. Is there a possibility to live even *slightly* more in tune with your internal clock? What changes will that require? Major ones? Small ones? What is the most important thing for you right now?

When we start making these changes, little by little, we notice how our lifeforce, prana, starts flowing more freely. According to traditional Chinese medicine, the body will die once we run out of *qi,* the vital force. We must personally want to make changes in our lives. A disease provides us with an amazing spiritual opportunity for this.

Work is not supposed to completely drain us. If every morning you leave for work feeling heavy and reluctant or your work brings you no joy, I would seriously recommend thinking about how you could change your life to allow your personality to flourish and feel well. The same goes for interpersonal relationships. Relationships are not supposed to drain our energy; rather, they should lift our spirits. The relationships we have with our partner and friends are supposed to give us energy, not rob us of it. When you look at your friendships, can you detect any that are draining your energy—ones that you are perhaps only holding onto out of habit? Or maybe because you are being too "nice"?

When we let our mind find peace, it will inform us what it will take for us to heal. The studies examining people who have experienced unexpected remission have found that what all these individuals have in common is a belief in their body's inherent and intuitive knowledge of what it needs for healing.

If something in your life makes you feel your internal alarm going off, feels that it is not right or good for you, you should always listen to this feeling, or at least take some time in making a major decision. Trust your intuition.

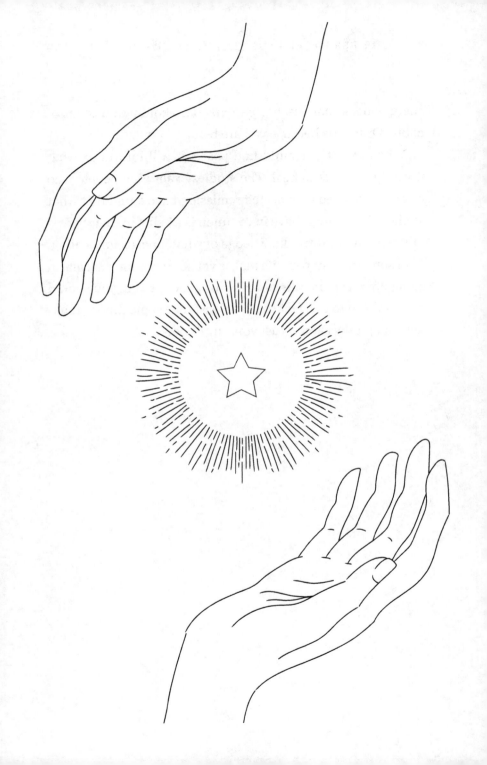

DHARMA CODE: YOUR
LIFE'S MISSION

E very day, I receive phone calls and emails from people
with cancer. I feel my mission in life is to help, encourage, and give hope to others. When people ask me "What have
you done to promote your healing?" I simply cannot give them
an answer that would fit into a single email or telephone con-
versation. I am also a firm believer of individuality on every
person's healing path.

When people fall ill or go through some other traumatic
experience, the things that happen to them are fairly similar.
We start paying attention to what we really want from life.
How do we wish to spend the time we have here on earth?
Who are the people who give us more strength? And who are
the people and things that deplete strength?

I have always found it important that I enjoy my job. I have
always been a true "free spirit," an artist, a free soul. I could

never fit into any sort of a ready-made mold; instead, my life has been highly varying and irregular. That especially applied to my work. I have had such varied jobs: I have been a flight attendant, a project manager at an event production company, a coder of electronic music, a DJ, a waitress in Spain, an au pair in Sweden, a journalist, and a TV announcer.

I remember once having to list my most important personal values on paper when participating in a life coach training. I had never thought about this before. All I had been doing was sprinting through life without giving anything a deeper thought. I remember seeing others write down words on their pieces of paper while my mind drew a blank. In the end, I only wrote down one word: *freedom.*

Now, as a result of my illness, it has felt as if all my life experience, life skills coaching studies, and travels were interconnected. My life's mission has been crystallized. While I am still interested in hosting, I also organize well-being events and give lectures to companies. I also set up yoga, welfare, and nature adventure retreats around the world. That spark for helping others that has always been in me remains. It is like a seed that has been given a chance to grow, little by little.

Now I get to share everything my whole life and this illness has brought me. It has changed me. I think about things more profoundly than ever before. I feel more deeply. I continue to be immersed in other people's emotions too much. I continue to struggle with setting boundaries. Nevertheless, I have become better at it. And while I am already much better at saying no to things, it continues to be a challenge. Apparently, I am still going to have to hit my head against a wall a few more times.

Physically, my illness has left minor memory traces in my body. My coordination is bit poorer. My right leg is a bit "loose" below the knee. Sometimes in yoga, I have to pay attention to what my right leg is doing as I cannot feel it as strongly as before.

On the other hand, I have never felt healthier and more balanced than now. I now understand what health means. I no longer take health for granted, but cherish it with my everyday choices instead.

I was able to get my driver's license back. In the spring of 2015, I walked into a local driving school and asked them to give me driving lessons. The weakness in my coordination and loss of feeling in my leg are what make driving difficult for me. I have so much sympathy for my driving teacher, who was patient enough to believe that things would work out for me. We just kept repeating, repeating, repeating. Your brain will eventually learn things as long as you keep practicing enough. And what do you know—even though I struggled with starting my car at first, I was able to train my brain to drive again as a result of persistent practice. Now driving feels natural to me. And I am a good driver, to boot!

None of these minor physical hindrances are perceptible to outsiders. I live a perfectly "normal" life of a "healthy person." My son Rene is, at 18, officially an adult by Finnish standards—and so tall his head nearly scrapes the ceiling! His brother Nooa has grown to love the skateboard, so I seldom see him indoors. They are happy, active teenagers. Jussi and I separated—amicably—a few years back, but he is still an important part of our family and my best friend, and we parent our boys together. As this relationship grows into its new form, I find how uniquely significant each relationship is to my own growth and sense of wellness. Every friendship, every connection matters. I continue my work to elevate the cause of human rights—especially the rights of children. I feel a great sense of humility and gratitude for being able to still be part of all the lives my life has touched. At least for today, I get to live! Hopefully still for a long time to come.

It has been years since my last epileptic seizure. I continue to obediently take a small dose of epilepsy medication every day. I hope that someday, I will be able to ditch the medication altogether. That day is already very near.

I remember my five-year anniversary of cancer-free MRI scans. That is considered an official marker after which you can pretty much count yourself as a healthy person. I remember asking my cancer specialist, Hanna: "Are you going to give me that "bill of health" that was promised to me?" While these five years do not guarantee anything, passing the mark has nevertheless slightly increased my mental calmness and faith in being able to heal after all.

I crossed one major milestone.

These days, I have a head MRI once per year. I still get slightly anxious about them.

Joy, laughter and humor are all very important to me. I cherish joy. Life must not be excessively boring and laborious.

I believe we all have our own "dharma code." That one thing your soul is screaming for. It does not have to be your job. It can be something else like turning your love for animals into spending your leisure time training dogs and volunteering as a dog trainer. Or it could take shape as an art exhibition, starting an orphanage in Nepal, taking in a foster child, volunteering with older people. It can be anything! I believe we all have a purpose—at least the small seed or a sapling of one. For many, purpose is dormant. When you're pulled out of regular everyday life, you start to look at things from a different perspective and restructure with the larger picture in mind.

Through crisis (wouldn't it be nice if it *wasn't* crisis, though?!) or some big life event, you start to find purpose—it starts to emerge and become more clear.

In early spring 2016, I was lecturing with my dear friend, stress coach Miia Huitti, at an event for supporting people with cancer here in Finland. I gave a lecture on my cancer journey and what I had done for my healing, while Miia spoke about the effects of stress on illnesses. We had astonishing chemistry and shared the idea that everything is possible if we are brave enough to believe it. Bravery and courage is something we have in spades.

On our drive back, I spoke with Miia about how this is exactly what people with cancer need: knowledge, hope, and positive peer support. It is not right that a person with cancer has to go abroad to seek holistic help. Or they get told in a hospital that their diet does not matter. Or people with cancer are told not to take CAM therapies, also known as complementary therapies. It is not right people with cancer are not given hope.

I wish I would have received peer support, particularly at the initial stages of my illness. Positive peer support. Looking back I wish right from the get-go, I would have had information about nutrition and its significance to healing. I would have asked for emotional support. I would've sought complementary therapies allowing me to completely relax my body after all the tension, worry and stress. I would have asked for support in finding out how I could personally affect my healing. Instead, I had to seek out all of this information by myself, gathering bits of knowledge from here and there. I had to listen to my intuition: what resonated with me and what did not. I had to personally find out about things, and spend hours online, reading and studying. If only someone had provided me with all of this from the start.

Cancer does not only affect the patient, but the whole family. It is extremely important that family members are taken into account, and that they get the support and help they need. Family members can't talk about everything to the patient. They also need someone to talk to, and decompress by opening up. Sometimes caretakers ignore their own needs in the process of caretaking and get burnt out. Then *they* get ill!

On our drive, we decided that we would create this package that would provide people with holistic help, including all the things I found to be extremely important on my journey. We wanted to create something accessible which everyone could participate in: a program where medical treatments are supported with gentle therapies affecting the body and mind, a lot of information about diet, and positive peer support. Support and information about the change each newly-diagnosed person is going to face. Our team includes doctors, functional dietitians, phytotherapists, and people who have healed from cancer.

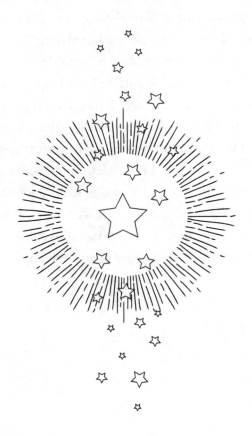

COMBINING MEDICINE WITH COMPLEMENTARY THERAPIES (CAM)

O nce I started having a clearer idea that my lifework would involve helping other people with cancer, my greatest mission took a clear form: to advocate that medical treatments, complementary therapies, and diet go hand in hand.

It is not right for patients to have to "hide" the fact that they are supporting their medical treatment with therapies such as acupuncture, mind-body therapies, or reflexology, if the patients feel that they are getting benefits from these types of care. I see red when medical professionals refer to them as "alternative therapies" or "pseudo-medicine." The majority of patients do not refuse the medical treatments offered to them. But a large share of them support these treatments with complementary therapies. Pseudomedicine refers to something that is quite frankly bogus, total nonsense. That is not what we are dealing with here.

The purpose of complementary therapies is to *complement* medical treatment. They are not used as a replacement for surgery, radiotherapy, or cytostatic agents. As I have noted previously in this book, it is extremely important for us to take some responsibility for our treatments and our health. We, the patients, want to be involved in planning the right treatment for us and to also take some personal responsibility for it.

I am interested in the ways and forms of help people have found beneficial. I am less interested in scientific studies, which contain lots and lots of views in favor and against certain things. It's important to always read scientific studies with a critical view: who or what organization funded the study? Who does the study benefit? Is it a pharmaceutical company? Is it a major oil corporation? What I want to know is what experiences people have had, what are the things they have found helpful in recovering from their diseases. I strongly believe that doctors' attitudes towards complementary therapies are becoming increasingly positive.

The complementary therapies I have used include acupuncture, craniosacral therapy, reflexology, aromatherapy, phytotherapy (herbal medicine), and many mind–body therapies. I know that these complementary therapies have been helpful for me, and I do not need this view to be supported by boring research findings, even though numerous studies show the efficacy of these therapies.

It is not enough to merely focus on the body while ignoring the health of the mind. Every person is a whole. Even though medicine is making constant progress and there is increasing understanding of the treatment of diseases, society continues to get sicker. People suffer from stress, obesity, high blood pressure, burnout, depression, diabetes. There is also a group of people inhabiting a space between sickness and health. They are not exactly ill, but are still unwell. They are not vibrant or balanced. Instead of pumping these people full of pills, introducing complementary therapies, emotional support, and dietary changes in their lives would be beneficial, rather than waiting until they are really, truly ill.

I witness the importance of holistic treatment for people as I lead my Nordic Guide to Healing Seminars and retreats. I have seen with my own eyes how people with cancer get immense strength from positive peer support, healthy diet supporting healing, experiences of cancer survivors, and mind–body therapies. All of these aspects contribute to healing. Peer support gives people hope that they, too, can recover from cancer.

One important part of healing involves releasing our emotional blocks and traumas. On this topic, I interviewed Professor Markku Partinen who has a PhD in medicine and surgery.

He explained to me how childhood traumas directly affect a person's immunity, therefore resulting in the onset of illness later in life. I believe this lies at the core of healing. A mental trauma, emotional stress, pent-up emotions, or emotional blocks that have turned into chronic stress in the body over time may not be visible from the outside. This phenomenon may also be fully unconscious. But our bodies are wise. The body will carry these things until they can become visible. In a way, the trauma or block will eventually force itself out of the body. For us, it will be apparent in the form of a physical disease that actually contains the emotional trauma. We can take this opportunity for beginning the healing process —once that thing you have been carrying with you all along has become visible.

Your resilience, i.e. mental capacity for recovery, is helpful in surviving a serious illness, as with any other adversities in life. Resilience is a psychological characteristic, which some of us possess more than others. Some of us are able to survive many severe crises while others fail to cope with minor hardships.

A person's resilience keeps transforming throughout their entire life. Different factors, including upbringing and biological traits, affect resilience. Even at the level of genes, we differ in terms of our sensitivity to the impact of our environment. Resilience may also be constructed in the individual's personal experiences by an interaction between positive and negative factors emerging from their community and environment.

The good news, however, is that resilience is not a fixed characteristic; instead, it is a skill everyone can practice. Resilience grows as we age and develop skills making it easier for us to encounter adversities. These include problem-solving skills, flexibility, self-regulation ability, and optimism. When you are living through a difficult time, hearing other people's stories of survival may also help you feel that if others have survived the same thing, you will too.

Humor also plays an important role in healing. Many friends have asked me if I find it difficult to constantly listen to the stories of people with cancer. I do not think I have ever laughed as heartily as I have with other people affected by cancer, who I consider My People. The sense of community I have felt with others when looking at a line of wigs in a sauna locker room is hard to put into words. It is extremely important to find joy and laughter, even when we are struck by illness.

I hope the medicine of the future will pay more attention to people as a whole. We need a large group of people who believe in our ability to heal to support the medical treatments. I also hope we will get permission to use the complementary therapies we believe will help us. I hope these complementary therapies will be covered by insurance or state care, and patients do not have to pay out of pocket for these. I hope we are guided in finding a diet that promotes our healing.

Most importantly, I wish for hope. Future medicine should put increased attention towards listening to patients' needs and wishes. Care must be patient-directed. This should involve giving us our diagnoses realistically, but still keeping our hopes up, no matter how poor our prospects. And doctors should encourage patients to take personal responsibility for their own healing.

In the future, hospitals should serve food that *supports* patients' healing process.

Patients' wishes should be heard, taking into account their hopes for the next move and how they are feeling in the middle of all that they are going through.

Patients' families should be heard. They should also be asked about how they are doing, and how they wish to be helped and supported.

Cancer survivors should be heard. They should be asked about what they have done to promote their recovery and which aspects they believe have helped them recover.

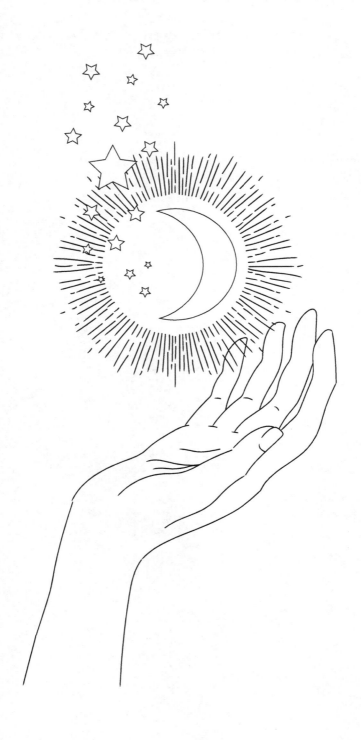

CONCLUSION

You do not beat cancer. This is not a competition with losers and winners. This is not a battle. This is simply a part of life. The idea a person "loses the cancer battle" for "not having enough fight left in them" does not sound right to me. It is another low blow for anyone who has lost a loved one to cancer. There are many people who I am sure have done all they can but have still passed away. We cannot say these people have "lost the fight". We must be humbled by this important and serious matter. No one knows what tomorrow will bring. I get to be grateful for each day I am here. Today, I am feeling well. Today, I am healthy.

I am not fighting cancer. I am living with it. I am trying to learn from it. What has it come to teach me? What have I not learned yet? What must I change in my life and how do I have to change so I can heal? What do I think my body will need to heal?

I see my tumor as my friend. A little friend who has come here to teach me to live a better life, a life that looks like me— and, most importantly, conforms to my personal values. I pay close attention to this little guy. Which turn should I take? Which path have I been on so many times I can abandon it for good? Which things have I said "YES" to before when I should have said "NO"? What are the things that simply do not serve me at this point?

If I am letting something new into my life, I have to get rid of something old. This allows me to keep things in balance and not overburden myself with more and more duties.

I hope I have succeeded in telling you my story in the most simple and down-to-earth way possible. I want to give you hope and courage. Keep having faith and trusting the power of your body. You already have all that you need.

Take responsibility for your healing. You are the CEO of your healing process.

ACKNOWLEDGEMENTS

A warm thank you to everyone who has walked on this path with me.

THANK YOU:

Rene and Nooa—words will not suffice. You are the greatest loves of my life.

Jussi—for your calmness, strength, and for carrying me

Mother and father—for your practical help, trust and belief in my healing

My sisters Kikka and Kati and all my dear relatives and friends

My brain surgeon Timo Tähtinen—the only person who has literally been inside my head. And saved my life. Twice.

My cancer specialists at Tampere University hospital

Chief Physician in Neurology Jukka Peltola

My teams at the Viisas Elämä and Nordic Wisdom publishing companies

The Old Gang—You are part of my family

HealthSummit Finland team

"The first aid team" on my home street

Yaron Butterfield

Microbiologist Elias Hakalehto, PhD

Professor Olli Polo, PhD

Professor Dominique Syrel

Markku Partinen, PhD, Specialist in Neurology

For the English edition, a big thank you to our amazing team: Harri Nyman, Julia Alakulju, Elisa Wulff, Cyan, Jaana Virronen, Ann Humphreys

And biggest thanks of all to my agent and a good friend Bhakti Kulmala - without your help and support this would have not been published in English. You are amazing!

Finally, to everyone affected by cancer.
You are all part of my Healing Circle.

Sources & Inspirations

- Eat to Beat Cancer, eattobeat.org
- Eckhart Tolle, The Power of Now
- The Gerson Institute, gerson.org
- Kelly Turner, Radical Remission: Surviving Cancer Against All Odds
- Richard Beliveau & Denis Gingras, Foods to Fight Cancer
- Anita Moorjani, Dying to Be Me: My Journey from Cancer, to Near Death, to True Healing
- Dr. David Servan-Schreiber, Anticancer—A New Way of Life
- Michael Greger & Gene Stone, How Not to Die
- Ben Williams, Surviving Terminal Cancer
- Jane Plant, Your Life In Your Hands
- Donna Eden, Energy Medicine: How to Use Your Body's Energies for Optimum Health and Vitality
- Kris Carr, Crazy Sexy Kitchen
- Andrew Cooper, Juiceman
- Henry March, Admissions: A Life in Brain Surgery

- Janesh Vaidya, Boost Your Immune Power with Ayurveda: Simple Lifestyle Adjustments to Balance the Elements in the Body & Mind
- Lissa Rankin, Mind Over Medicine
- Louise Hay, You Can Heal Your Life
- HEAL documentary
- National Cancer Institute, cancer.gov
- NCBI medical publications, ncbi.nlm.nih.gov
- Rod Styker, The Four Desires
- The Truth about Cancer, thetruthaboutcancer.com

Connect with Karita

nordicguidetohealing.com

NordicWisdom.com

Nordic Wisdom is a publishing house from Finland with a focus on Nordic myths, wellbeing, and way of life.
Discover that one thing that changes everything.

CPSIA information can be obtained
at www.ICGtesting.com
Printed in the USA
BVHW080851070921
616214BV00014B/746